MASSAGE

~ FOR BEGINNERS~
2022

THE BEST GUIDE TO RELAXATION AND PAIN RELIEF

CONTENTS

1 INTRODUCTION

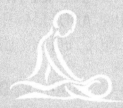

You can't stop the waves, but you can learn to swim.

JON KABAT ZINN

WELCOME

I HAVE ALWAYS BEEN INTERESTED IN MASSAGE THERAPY AS A WAY TO FEEL BETTER AND MORE CONNECTED WITH PEOPLE, AND I AM THRILLED TO BE ABLE TO SHARE MY KNOWLEDGE OF CLASSIC MASSAGE TECHNIQUES WITH YOU IN THIS BOOK.

THE MAGIC OF MASSAGE IS THAT IT CAN GUIDE A BODY TOWARD HEALING ITSELF. IT CAN HELP SOMEONE WHO IS SUFFERING TO FEEL BETTER THROUGHOUT THEIR HEALING PROCESS. MASSAGE BRINGS US BACK TO OURSELVES, REMINDING US TO LISTEN AND TO BREATHE, TO SLOW DOWN AND ACKNOWLEDGE PAIN AND TENSION, AND TO TAKE CARE OF OUR BODIES TENDERLY.

I GREW UP WITH SCOLIOSIS, AND REGULARLY EXPERIENCED THE FRUSTRATION AND STRESS OF CHRONIC PAIN. MY EARLIEST MEMORY OF MASSAGE IS OF MY MOTHER, A CLASSICALLY TRAINED PROFESSIONAL BALLERINA, WORKING ON MY SHOULDER PAIN USING KNEADING STROKES, WHICH GAVE ME SOME MUCH-NEEDED RELIEF. LATER, I WOULD GO ON TO TRADE BACK RUBS WITH FRIENDS, AND READ EVERY BOOK I COULD FIND ON THE SUBJECT OF MASSAGE.

I FIRST STUDIED MASSAGE FORMALLY IN THAILAND, BECOMING CERTIFIED IN THAI MASSAGE AT THE WAT PO SCHOOL IN BANGKOK. I IMMEDIATELY REALIZED THE BENEFITS AND JOY OF WORKING WITH MY HANDS AND WITH PEOPLE.

I CONTINUED MY EDUCATION AT THE SWEDISH INSTITUTE, AND BECAME LICENSED AS A MASSAGE THERAPIST IN NEW YORK, WHERE I PRACTICE TODAY. MY STUDIO COMBINES A MEDICALLY BASED MASSAGE PRACTICE WITH THE RELAXING ENVIRONMENT OF A HEALING SPACE, AND IT IS WONDERFUL PLACE TO BE: IT'S NOT WITH EVERY JOB THAT YOU GET TO BE THE BEST PART OF SOMEONE'S DAY, EVERY DAY.

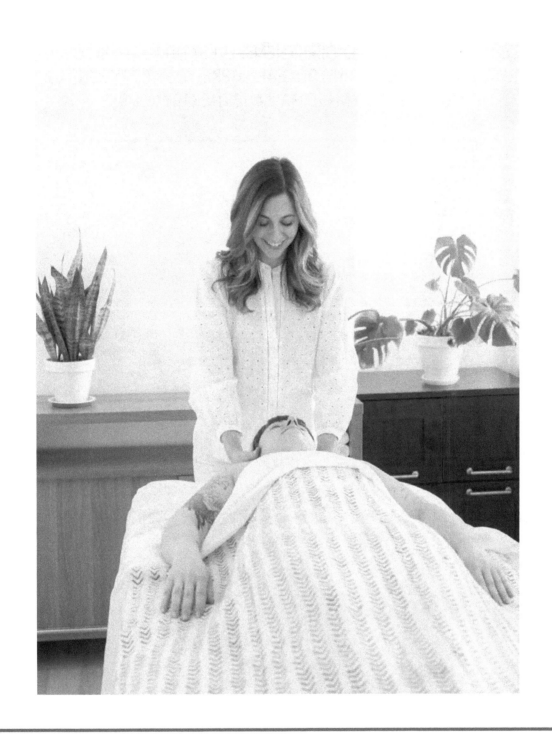

Disclaimer

UTILIZED AS A GIFT TO THE READERS THEMSELVES AND TO THEIR LOVED ONES. IF YOU ARE INSPIRED BY WHAT YOU LEARN HERE, YOU ARE ENCOURAGED TO JOIN AN ACCREDITED MASSAGE THERAPY COURSE.

A BRIEF HISTORY OF MASSAGE

Ancient civilizations dating back over 5,000 years have used massage for its healing properties.

3000BCE

The earliest mentions of massage were from India, in Ayurvedic texts and in oral history as early as 3000BCE.

|

2700BCE

In China, ancient texts describing medical massage, called Amma, appear in approximately 2700BCE.

|

2500BCE

Egyptian tomb paintings of people thought to be practicing massage date back to 2500BCE, and Egyptians are credited with creating the practice of reflexology.

|

1000BCE

Japanese monks studying Buddhism in China brought massage back to Japan around 1000BCE, creating Shiatsu.

|

500BCE

Hippocrates prescribed friction massage around the 5th century BCE, to help heal injuries.

|

1800AD

Europe began recognizing massage and its benefits in the 18th century, when the Swedish physician P. H. Ling used massage therapy to treat and prevent injuries for his gymnastic movement practice, popularizing massage in the west and creating an awareness of Swedish massage, which is the focus of this book.

|

TODAY

In modern times, massage is used for stress reduction, relaxation, injury recovery, and to feel more connected and grounded.

THE BENEFITS OF MASSAGE

The benefits of massage are immeasurable, as they reach the physical body, mind, and spirit. As humans, the mind–body connection is extremely powerful. There's no better way of accessing that connection than through physical touch, provided with dignity and respect. A better-feeling body leads to a better-feeling mind.

Practicing massage is a wonderful way to connect, to the receiver and to yourself. It builds trust and fosters a feeling of wellbeing for both the massage provider and the receiver in the work.

People seek out massage for many different reasons, including shoulder tension, back pain, joint stiffness, neck issues, jaw pain, headaches, sports injuries, arthritis, insomnia, carpal tunnel syndrome, menstrual cramps, fibromyalgia, and mood disorders such as anxiety and depression.

We know that any injury or issue is made significantly worse by stress, and massage is an excellent tool for stress reduction.

★

Massage is an important part of self-care, and works best when combined with a healthy regimen of stretching and strengthening exercises.

Massage Can Help to ...

RELIEVE PAIN

RELIEVE ANXIETY

REDUCE STRESS

REDUCE SYMPTOMS OF DEPRESSION

EASE MUSCLE TENSION

IMPROVE CIRCULATION

IMPROVE SLEEP

INCREASE RANGE OF MOTION

INCREASE FLEXIBILITY

FOSTER A FEELING OF BALANCE

FOSTER A SENSE OF CONNECTION

FOSTER A SENSE OF WELLBEING

ENCOURAGE DEEP RELAXATION

ABOUT THIS BOOK

This contemporary take on a traditional practice makes massage accessible to a new generation of readers.

Planning Your Session

SHOWN HERE

Here you will learn about the types of strokes and how to apply them, as well as how to plan a session, from setting the mood to understanding what is happening beneath the fingertips.

Self-Care for the Provider

SHOWN HERE

The massage provider must look after themselves as well as the receiver, so here you will learn basic preparatory stretches and how to use your body comfortably during a massage.

3

Getting to Work

SHOWN HERE

This chapter teaches you everything you need to know to give a phenomenal, step-by-step massage rooted in anatomy and physiology. You will learn how to massage each area of the body and how to address the major muscle groups.

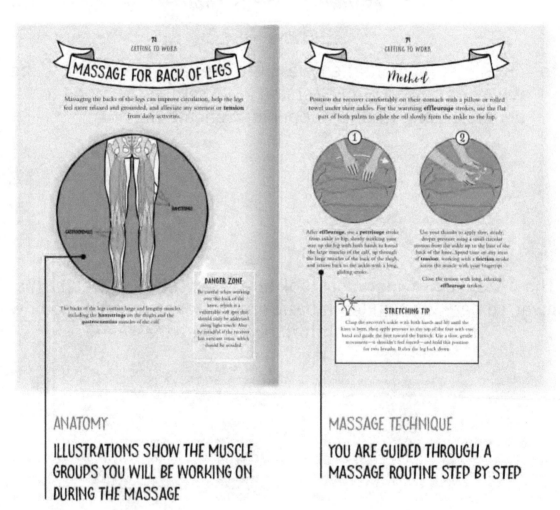

ANATOMY

ILLUSTRATIONS SHOW THE MUSCLE GROUPS YOU WILL BE WORKING ON DURING THE MASSAGE

MASSAGE TECHNIQUE

YOU ARE GUIDED THROUGH A MASSAGE ROUTINE STEP BY STEP

Treatment Plans

SHOWN HERE

This chapter explores various protocols for specific ailments. You will learn where to focus a massage to bring relief from symptoms such as headache, sinus congestion, and arthritis.

LABELS

NUMBERS AND ILLUSTRATIONS GUIDE YOU
THROUGH THE SPECIFIC PROTOCOLS

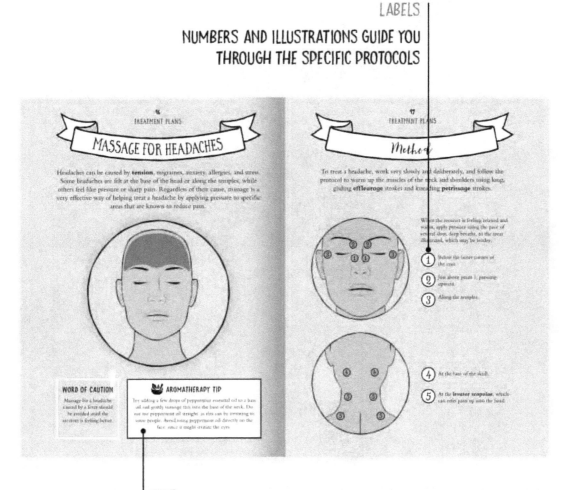

TIPS

EXTRA INFORMATION TO HELP BRING
RELIEF IS PROVIDED WHERE RELEVANT

5

Self-Massage

SHOWN HERE

This chapter shows you how you can effectively apply massage techniques to yourself, whether by hand or with the aid of a foam roller or tennis ball.

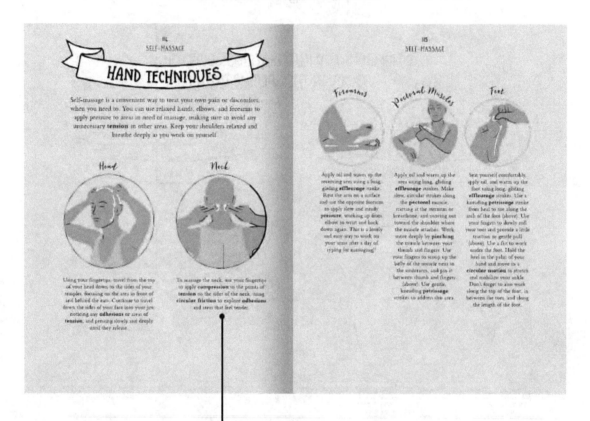

GUIDELINES

LEARN WHICH AREAS OF THE BODY
YOU CAN MASSAGE YOURSELF

2 PLANNING YOUR SESSION

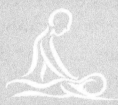

Breathe. Let go. And remind yourself that this very moment is the only one you know you have for sure.

OPRAH WINFREY

TYPES OF STROKES

There are seven different types of strokes used in a modern Swedish massage. This book will teach you about compression, the long, gliding strokes of effleurage, and the deep kneading strokes of petrissage. You'll be introduced to the muscle-tracing strokes of stripping, the therapeutic use of cross-fiber friction, the tone-producing stroke of tapotement, and the depth of trigger-point therapy for pain relief.

Compression

Compression strokes use the **flat part of the palms** to slowly introduce your touch and to warm up an area. This is a very **relaxing**, **pressing** stroke, where you slowly sink into the receiver as they exhale, moving **rhythmically with their breath** and easing up on the pressure with every inhale. Compression can be applied without oil, through sheets or clothing, and is useful if you're unable to work directly on the skin. More intense specific compression is used for Trigger-Point Therapy (see here).

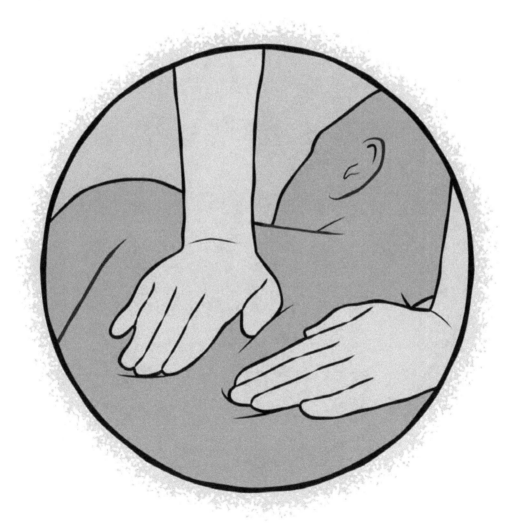

Effleurage

Effleurage strokes are **long**, **gliding**, **rhythmic**, and gentle. They are used in a traditional Swedish massage to introduce your touch to the receiver, and to spread out any oil or lotion. Use the **flat part of the palms**, keeping your hands relaxed, with **light to medium pressure**, while slowly gliding back and forth along the length of the muscles, making broad circles or slow waves. The slower your pace, the more relaxing the session will be.

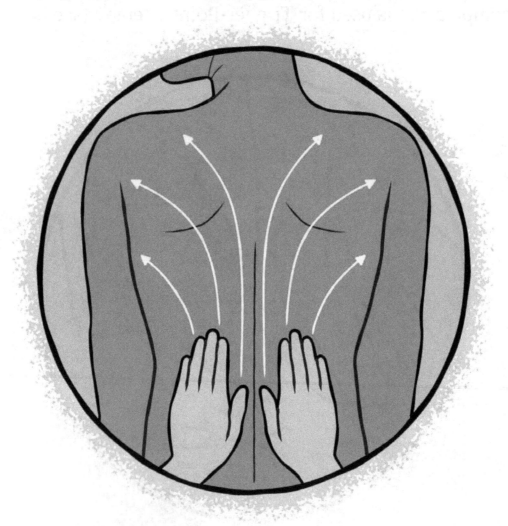

Petrissage

Petrissage follows effleurage, and uses **medium pressure** to **knead**, **pull**, **wring**, and **squeeze** the muscles. A **slow and steady rhythm** is used to bring circulation to an area, help the muscles to relax, and to warm up the body and prepare it for deeper work. Use the **whole part of the hand** to grasp and gently lift up the muscles, picking them up alternately between both hands. Use your thumbs to make slow, deep circles along the muscles.

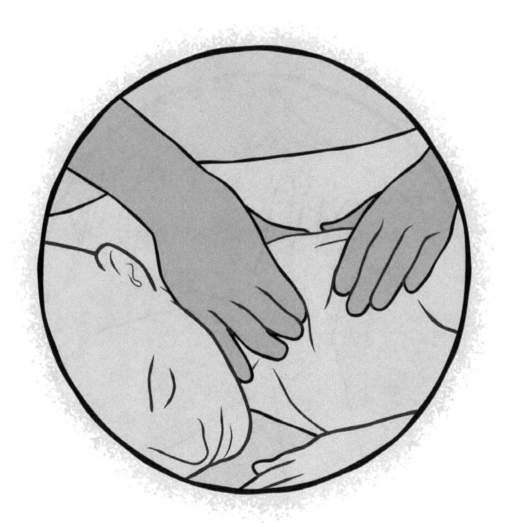

Stripping

A stripping stroke can be used along the **length of the muscle** for **deeper**, more focused work. Stripping can be done by using **fingertips**, **thumbs**, or the **heel of the hand** to **press deeply**, while moving slowly along the belly of the muscle, from one end of its attachment to the other. The intention is to feel for any areas of **tension**, or **adhesions** (see here) and, when you find them, to go deeply along them to help them release. Your hands should remain **firm but relaxed**.

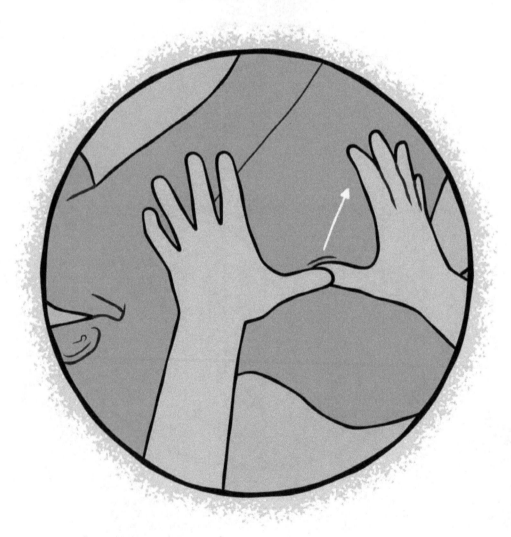

Cross-Fiber Friction

Cross-fiber friction is a **firm** and **deep** stroke performed against the **length of a muscle**, slowly going across the belly and the fibers, to help further reduce **adhesions**. The **fingertips or thumbs** are used to feel for areas in need of extra attention. Sink your fingers into the muscle and press firmly, moving slowly across the muscle fibers in a back and forth motion.

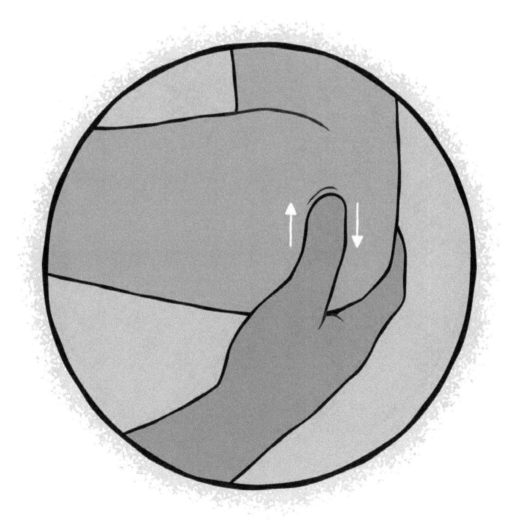

Tapotement

With tapotement, or pummeling, use **loosely clenched fists** or the **sides of your hands** to **bounce** off the flesh, **one hand after the other**. This is used especially in sports massage to warm up muscles. Your hands should be loose and relaxed as you rhythmically move up and down the body.

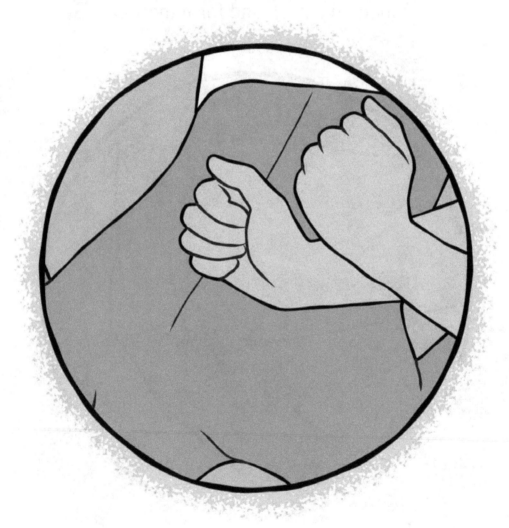

Trigger-Point Therapy

Trigger-point therapy works to **release bands of hyper-irritable muscle**. These spots create a pain-referral pattern that spreads to another area of the body. People tend to have trigger points in their shoulders or neck that cause tension headaches. To address a trigger point, **sink firmly into it**, holding the pressure for six to ten seconds, then gently release and use **circular strokes** to bring more circulation.

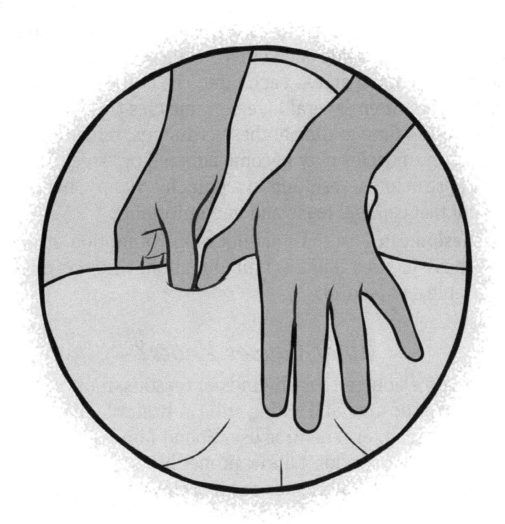

KNOTS

A knot is a hard, lumpy feeling in a muscle. The word "knot" is a misnomer, as muscles aren't literally tangled up. Instead, the muscle fibers start to stick together, forming an adhesion.

Crisscross Muscles

Our muscles are layered and oriented in many different directions. These layers cross each other at various angles. Think of some as parallel, running alongside each other, while others are perpendicular, running across each other. To complicate matters further, there are often several layers of muscles right on top of each other. From time to time at these crossings, rather than gliding past each other, muscles may become adhered or "stuck" to their surrounding structures, resulting in a crunchy, lumpy, hard, and painful spot that can feel tense and uncomfortable.

An **adhesion** can start to limit your range of motion, making it harder to move or stretch in a certain direction, which is often uncomfortable and painful.

What Causes Knots?

Muscles become adhered for all kinds of reasons, most commonly because of poor posture and sitting still (in front of a computer or at a desk) for too long, or repetitive use. Sound familiar? When we don't move around, we don't allow proper blood flow. Circulation is important because it lubricates our muscles, bringing fresh oxygen and nutrients. We aren't meant to be sedentary; our bodies need movement and action to stay healthy.

Another contributing factor to adhesions is dehydration. Coffee and alcohol are diuretics, and in order to stay well hydrated and in good shape, our bodies require water. Muscles are very spongy tissue, and need to stay well hydrated to perform at their best.

Injuries can also contribute to **adhesions**, and they are commonly found at points of scar tissue.

When You Find a Knot

When you think you've found a knot, check in with the receiver and ask them how that spot feels. If it's an area that they would like work done on, slowly sink your fingers in, making sure to check in regarding pressure (see Touch Pressure, shown here). The receiver should feel relief at having pressure placed on an area with a knot: the effect should feel like "delicious" pain, not scary pain. Use **cross-fiber** strokes or **circular friction** to address the area, always working within the pain tolerance of the receiver.

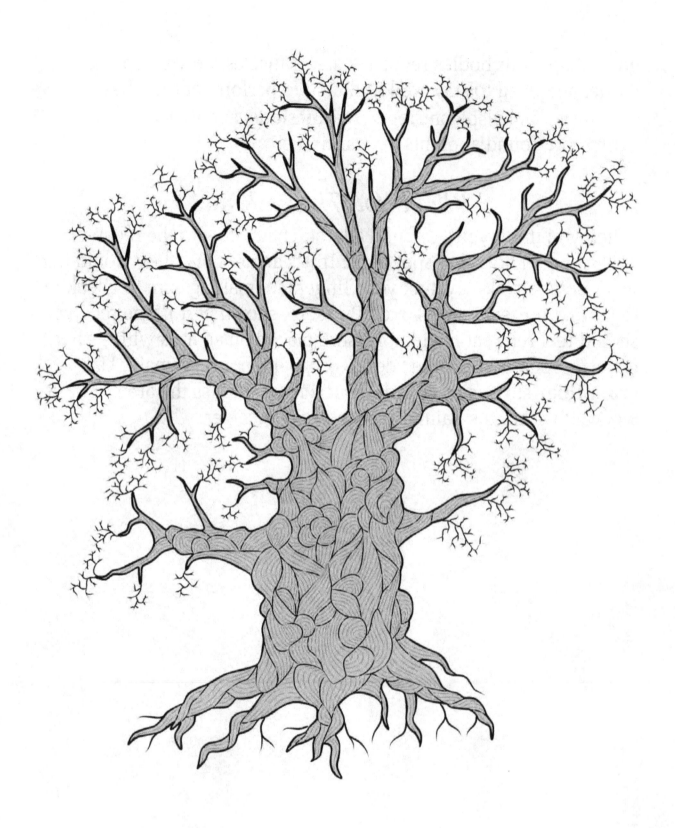

PAIN

We experience different types of pain, and the treatment massage can provide depends on the kind of pain being felt.

Muscle Pain

Muscular pain can feel **dull**, **achy**, **heavy**, and **sore**. **Massage is appropriate** for treating muscular pain.

Chronic Pain

Chronic pain is pain that **lasts for several months**, and can feel dull and achy or sharp and surprising, for stretches of time. Pain signals can remain active in our nervous system long after an injury has gone away. Examples of chronic pain include headaches, backaches, and arthritis. Massage can **be used safely** as a natural remedy to help **manage chronic pain**.

Acute Pain

Acute pain is **temporary, sudden, and surprising** in its onset. It often happens when we have an accident, burn, cut, broken bone, or injury. Because acute pain tends to involve inflammation, **massage is not appropriate** since it may cause more stress or pain.

Nerve Pain

Nerve pain is **sharp** and **shooting**, for example when you bump the ulnar nerve (sometimes called the funny bone) in your elbow. It can feel **electric**, or like pins and needles. **Massage is not appropriate** for nerve pain.

THE SKILL OF PALPATION

Palpation is the act of feeling what is happening underneath your fingertips. It's the difference between looking at a page with words on it and reading the page.

When we palpate well, we can respond to what we are feeling more efficiently. The best massage therapists are excellent practitioners of the skill of palpation. The best way of understanding what you are feeling when you place your hands on a receiver is to memorize the map of the body and its structures. Studying anatomy, as well as understanding the bony landmarks and the pathways of where each muscle begins and ends, will help you to recognize what you are feeling.

Experience the Feeling

To practice this skill, try placing a hair underneath a sheet of paper. Close your eyes and notice when you're able to feel the hair through the page. Add more sheets of paper to create an additional challenge for your senses and to heighten your skills.

TRIGGER POINTS

Trigger points are common spots in muscles that create a constellation of ache known as a pain-referral pattern. When a trigger point is compressed and stimulated, it is typical to feel pain in a remote area. For example, a trigger point in the shoulder may cause a headache or neck pain, especially when the point is stimulated.

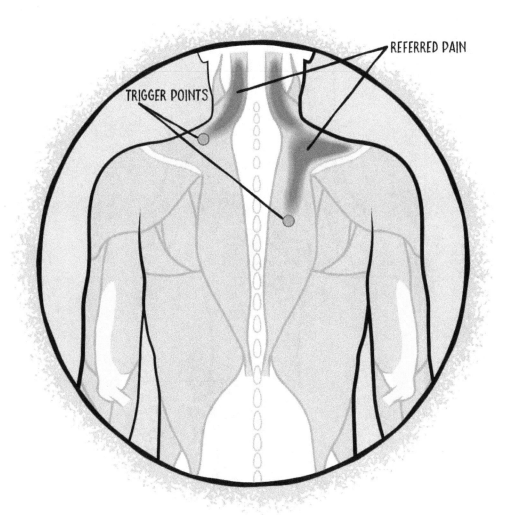

Referred Pain

A trigger point can feel a bit like a **bubble on water**. You'll notice that if you sink deeply into one, the receiver will often feel a referred pain in a distant area. Trigger points in the shoulders or neck, for example, can cause tension headaches. The intention of **compressing** a trigger point is to help it **release**, thereby taking it out of its contraction, **to alleviate pain**.

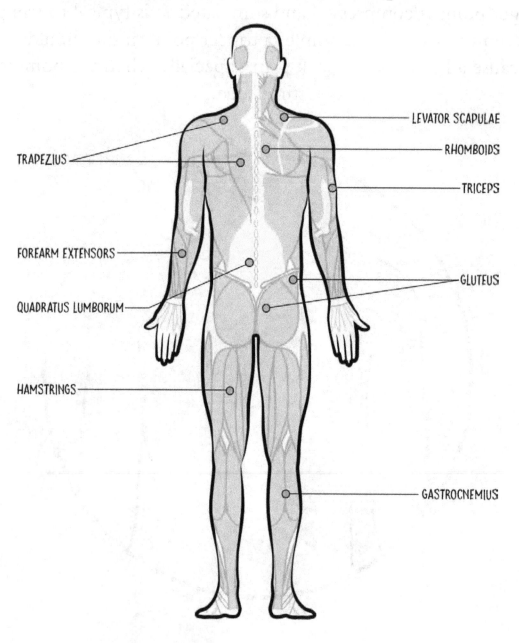

TRAPEZIUS

LEVATOR SCAPULAE

RHOMBOIDS

TRICEPS

FOREARM EXTENSORS

QUADRATUS LUMBORUM

GLUTEUS

HAMSTRINGS

GASTROCNEMIUS

Common trigger points

- Trapezius = shoulder and neck pain
- Levator scapulae = shoulder and neck pain
- Gluteus muscles = hip and lower back pain
- Forearm extensors = wrist and forearm pain
- Hamstrings = upper leg and hip pain
- Gastrocnemius = leg and ankle pain
- Rhomboids = shoulder pain
- Triceps = back of arm pain
- Quadratus lumborum = lower back pain

PREPARATION FOR MASSAGE

Preparation for massage is all about making sure the receiver is comfortable and able to relax in the environment. The massage provider should also be in the right frame of mind.

CHOOSE A TIME WHEN YOU WILL BOTH BE FREE FROM DISTRACTIONS
And can commit to relaxation and focus.

★

SET UP THE ROOM TO BE COMFORTABLE FOR THE RECEIVER
Making sure it is warm enough.

★

HAVE ALL OF YOUR SUPPLIES READY
Including a lotion or oil and any aromatherapy oils that you'd like to use.

★

HAVE PLENTY OF CUSHIONS OR PILLOWS AROUND FOR SUPPORT
As well as a towel or blanket in case the receiver gets cold.

★

DIM THE LIGHTS TO CREATE A RELAXING AND CALM ENVIRONMENT
You may want to use candles or incense to set the mood.

★

WASH YOUR HANDS BEFORE BEGINNING
And take a moment to center yourself.

Oils and Lotions

There are lots of options for lubrication for your session. Try experimenting with different lotions and oils until you find one that has a comfortable slip and glide.

Oils such as coconut, almond, grapeseed, or jojoba are a good slippery choice for lighter massage work. Water-based lotions or creams are better for deeper work because they are less slippery and can provide more traction, though they dry out more easily.

If you or the receiver has any allergies, make sure to choose a lubrication that doesn't trigger them. Always **warm** any oil or lotion **between your palms** by rubbing them briskly together. This is a far more relaxing way to apply lubricant than to squeeze it directly onto the receiver.

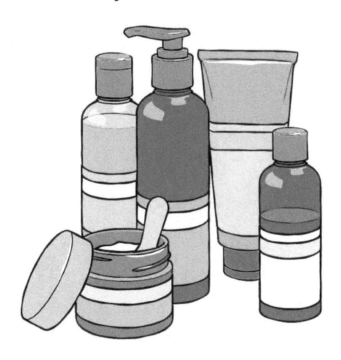

Aromatherapy

Adding a few drops of essential oil to a base oil can be a wonderful way to enhance the massage session. Essential oils should not be used alone, as some may irritate the skin if applied undiluted. Make sure to use a reputable brand, as some oils may include synthetics. Common essential oils used in massage include the following:

LAVENDER

Deeply relaxing
Effective for stress relief
Helps with sleep

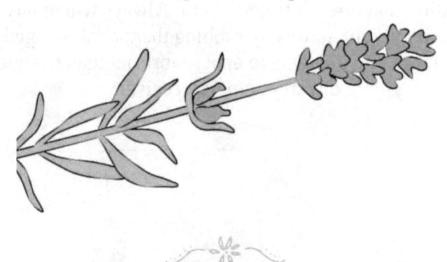

CHAMOMILE

Soothing
Promotes sleep
Good for deep relaxation

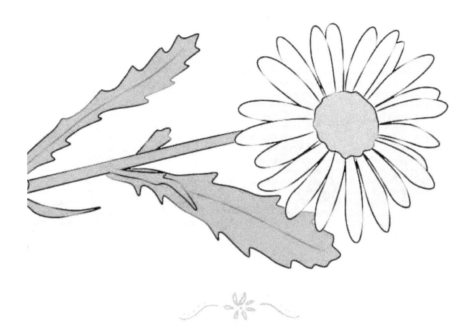

PEPPERMINT

Refreshing
Cooling
Excellent for headaches
Revives tired muscles

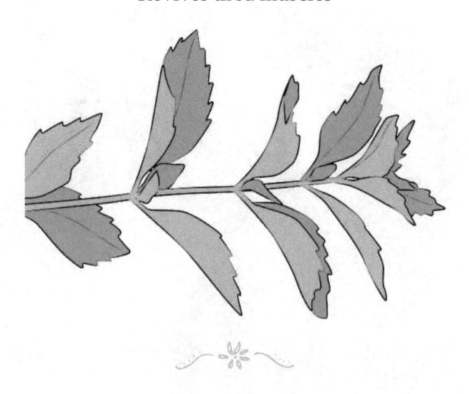

ROSEMARY

Helps to open up the lungs if the receiver has a cough

Can warm an area

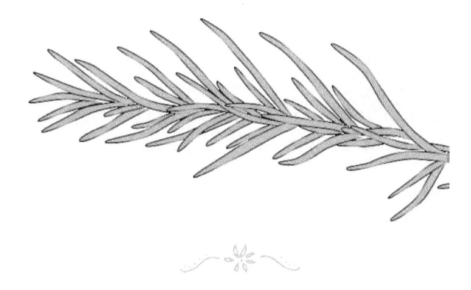

EUCALYPTUS

Helps treat congestion
Relieves aching muscles

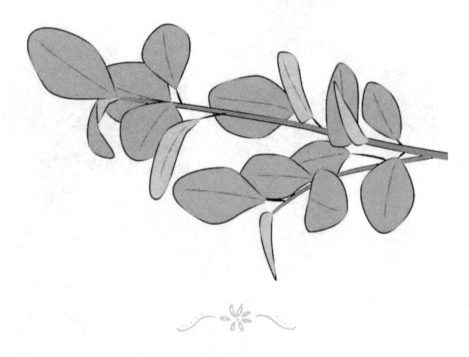

ORANGE

Refreshing and uplifting
Elevates mood

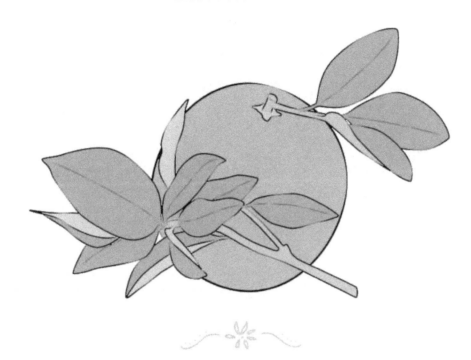

SANDALWOOD

Grounding Relaxing

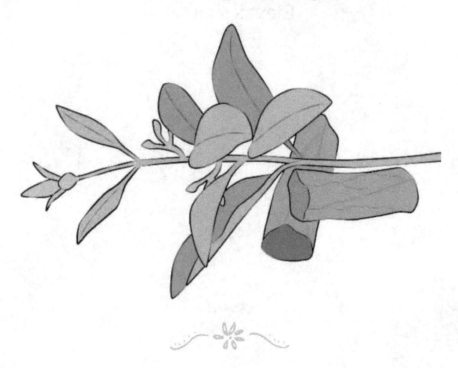

ROSE GERANIUM

Hormone balancing
Heart opening

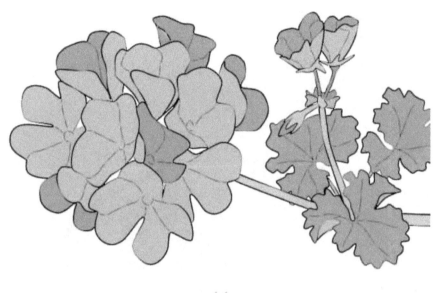

Applying Heat

Using heat during a session can add another deep level of relaxation and relief. Try warming up a therapeutic rice pack in the microwave, and carefully applying it at the start of a session (see here).

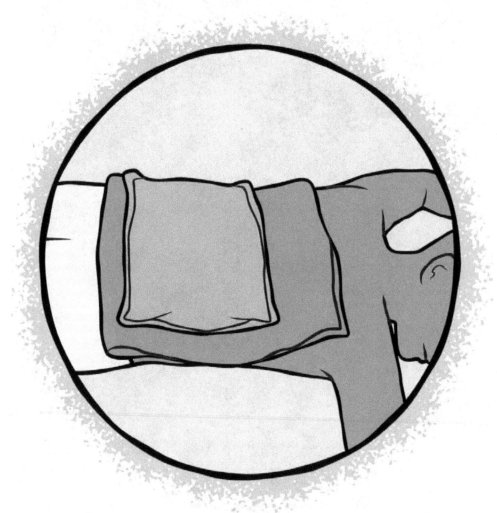

Laying Face Down

A heat pack may be applied to the neck, upper back, lower back, hips, thighs, or calves.

Laying Face Up

A heat pack can feel good underneath the neck, under the lower back, or on the abdomen for cramp relief.

PRECAUTIONS

There are certain situations in which massage should be avoided, including:

Do not massage areas of swelling, inflammation, or acute pain, or where there are varicose veins, open cuts or sores, or tumors or lumps.

★

Do not massage if the receiver has any signs of illness, such as fever, rash, nausea, vomiting, or is feeling generally unwell.

★

Avoid massage on any area of infectious skin conditions that may spread, including herpes or scabies.

★

Ask the receiver if they have any areas of bruising or pain, any allergies, and any history of injuries.

★

Do not work on anyone if they are intoxicated or under the influence of drugs or medication (such as pain medication) that compromises their ability to feel.

★

Do not apply these techniques during pregnancy. Please see a practitioner who specializes in prenatal massage during that time.

Consent

Make sure to always get informed consent before touching any area of the receiver and, should they feel uncomfortable or in pain, immediately stop what you're doing. Massage should always feel like "delicious pain," not scary pain.

COMMUNICATION

Communicating before, during, and after your session is incredibly important. The receiver should feel comfortable communicating their desires, boundaries, and needs, and should also feel safe in the knowledge that you will respond accordingly.

Before You Start

CHECK IN ABOUT ANY AREAS THAT THE RECEIVER WOULD LIKE YOU TO WORK ON, ASKING IN ADVANCE WHAT SPECIFICALLY THEY WOULD LIKE TO ADDRESS DURING THEIR SESSION.

Respect

FIND OUT IF THERE ARE ANY AREAS THAT THE RECEIVER DOES NOT WANT YOU TO TOUCH, AND ALWAYS RESPECT THEIR WISHES.

Touch Pressure

ASK THE RECEIVER ABOUT YOUR PRESSURE USING A ONE TO TEN SCALE, WITH ONE BEING TOO LIGHT AND TEN BEING TOO PAINFUL. THE GOAL SHOULD BE ABOUT A SIX OR SEVEN.

Visual Clues

STAY ALERT FOR VISUAL CUES FROM THE RECEIVER. THESE ARE NONVERBAL WAYS THAT THEY MAY BE COMMUNICATING DISCOMFORT, SUCH AS FACIAL EXPRESSIONS, CURLING OF TOES, TENSING UP, OR SHRUGGING THEIR SHOULDERS.

After

AFTER THE CLOSE OF THE SESSION (SEE HERE), ASK THE RECEIVER IF THEY HAVE ANY QUESTIONS OR CONCERNS.

3 SELF-CARE FOR THE PROVIDER

When you stretch, you open up space. This is physically true, and emotionally true. When you physically stretch, you create and allow for greater movement, greater vulnerability, and more growth.

KATE BARTOLOTTA

STRETCHES

Self-care is important for the massage provider in order to build up endurance and avoid injury while massaging. Warm up and stretch before and after your session, and keep hydrated by drinking water. Always circle your wrists and shake out your hands before and after the massage. Before stretching, gently warm up the muscles with some physical activity.

Arm Extenser Stretch

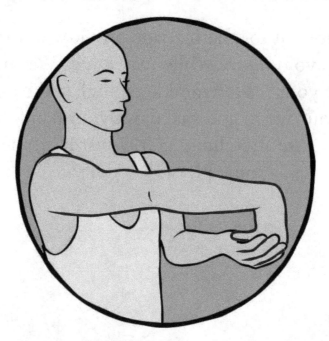

To stretch the extensors of the forearm (see here), hold your arm out straight in front of you and bend the hand palm-side down, relaxing the muscles. Make sure to keep your shoulders relaxed. Repeat on the other arm.

Arm Flexer Stretch

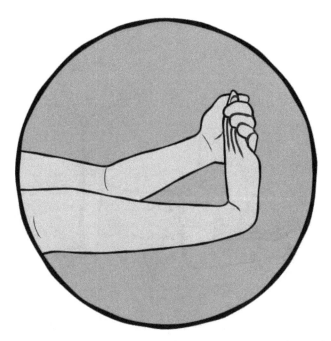

To stretch the wrists and flexors of the forearm (see here), hold your arm out straight in front of you and gently apply pressure to the fingertips, pulling them back toward your body. Use gentle pressure and slow movements. Repeat on the other arm.

Back Stretch

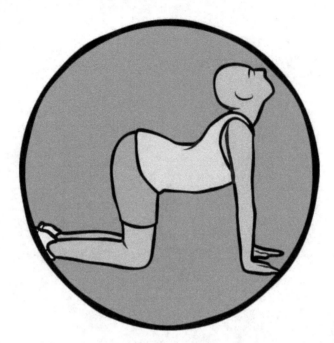

On your hands and knees, arch your spine while bringing your head and hips toward the sky, then reverse the stretch, raising your back into a rounded curve. Hold each pose for several deep breaths.

Hip and Gluteal Stretch

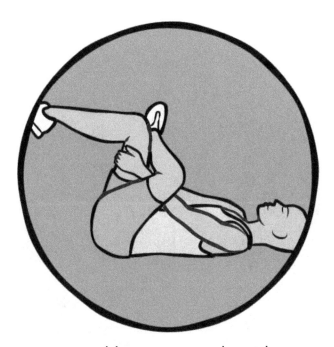

On your back, cross your ankle over your bent knee and reach through your legs to grasp your hands behind the free leg, pulling it toward your chest. Hold for several deep breaths, allowing the upper body to relax. Repeat on the other leg.

Shoulder and neck Stretches

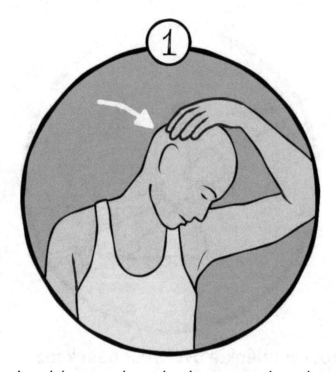

To stretch your shoulders and neck, sit on one hand and use the other one to gently maneuver the head toward the shoulder. Relax the tops of your shoulders as you apply slow and gentle pressure. Hold the pose for several deep breaths. Repeat on the other side.

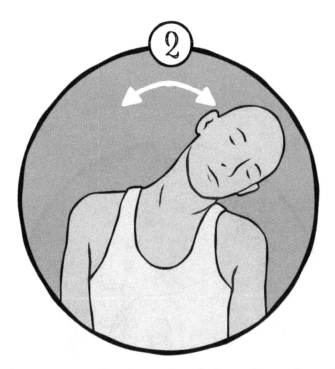

To gently stretch your neck, sit on both hands, palms face up, to lock your shoulders into place. Gently maneuver your ear toward one shoulder, then the other, holding each position for a few deep breaths. Make sure to keep your shoulders relaxed.

Chest Stretch

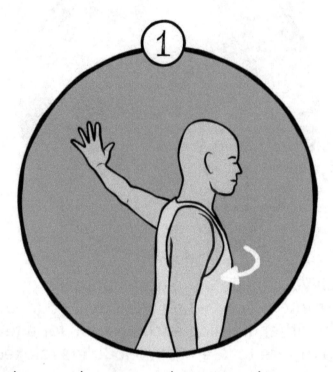

To stretch your chest and open up the arms, place your hand firmly on a wall with the arm outstretched, and slowly turn your body away from the wall. Take several deep breaths.

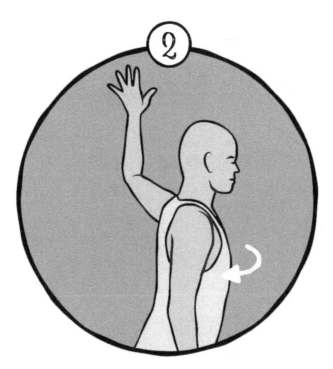

Repeat the same movement, but change your hand position so it is higher and lower in order to target different areas of the pectoral muscles. Repeat with the other arm on the wall.

ERGONOMICS DURING A SESSION

It's important to be mindful of the way your body is positioned and the way you move while giving a massage. Using good posture and body mechanics will help you to work with less physical discomfort and prevent injuries.

Distance

MAKE SURE THAT THERE IS ENOUGH DISTANCE BETWEEN YOU AND THE RECEIVER TO ALLOW YOU TO LEAN INTO THEM, RATHER THAN PRESSING WITH FORCE.

DO YOUR STRETCHES (SEE HERE).

Height

IF THE RECEIVER IS LYING DOWN, OR SEATED, POSITION THEM LOWER THAN YOU TO USE HEIGHT TO YOUR ADVANTAGE IN APPLYING PRESSURE.

Share the Load

DON'T MAKE YOUR FINGERTIPS DO ALL THE WORK. REMEMBER TO USE YOUR FOREARM, RELAXED FIST, OR A FLAT PALM WHERE POSSIBLE TO LEAN AND CREATE PRESSURE.

Good Practice

WHEN WORKING WITH YOUR HANDS, KEEP YOUR FINGERS RELAXED, YOUR SHOULDERS LOOSE AND DOWN, AND RELEASE ANY TENSION IN YOUR BODY.

Slow is Good

WORKING SLOWLY MEANS YOU CARRY OUT LESS REPETITIVE WORK THAN IF YOU WERE TO HASTEN YOUR SPEED, AND THE RECEIVER WILL FEEL MORE RELAXED, TOO.

Breathe

BE AWARE OF THE RISE AND FALL OF YOUR BREATH. THE RECEIVER'S BREATH MAY START TO SYNC WITH YOUR OWN. USE SLOW INHALATIONS AND LONGER, DEEPER EXHALATIONS TO ENCOURAGE THEM TO RELAX.

YOU ARE A HAPPY MASSAGE PROVIDER.

4 GETTING TO WORK

There is no exercise better for the heart than reaching down and lifting people up.

JOHN HOLMES

POSITIONING FOR COMFORT

The receiver should be comfortable enough to nod off during the massage session: this means using lots of pillows, towels, and blankets for support. If you don't have a massage table, a bed or sofa both work well.

Position Face Down

To position the receiver ergonomically when they are laying on their stomach, make sure they are supported under the head and ankles, allowing the legs to be straight with the feet raised. Place pillows or rolled towels under the head and ankles.

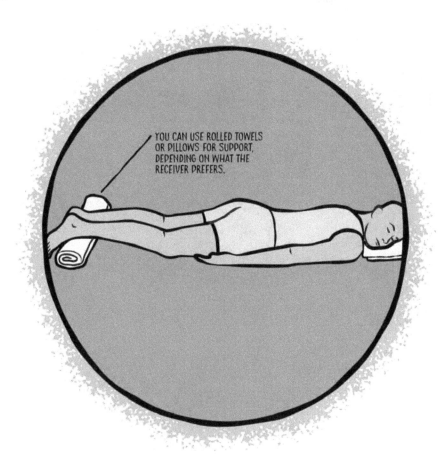

YOU CAN USE ROLLED TOWELS OR PILLOWS FOR SUPPORT, DEPENDING ON WHAT THE RECEIVER PREFERS.

Position Face Up

When the receiver is laying on their back, place extra pillows underneath the knees. This supports the neck and lower back without any added strain, and is very relaxing for anyone experiencing back pain.

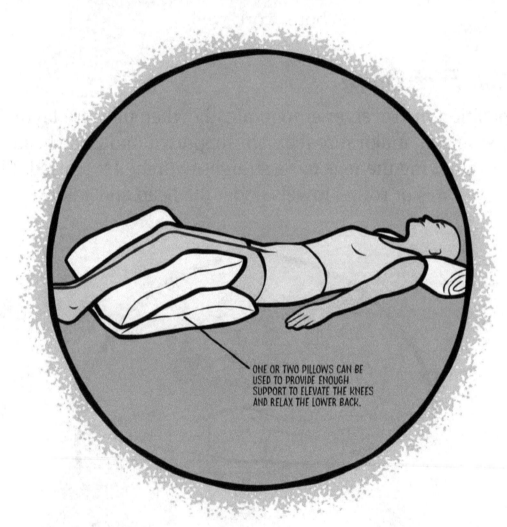

ONE OR TWO PILLOWS CAN BE USED TO PROVIDE ENOUGH SUPPORT TO ELEVATE THE KNEES AND RELAX THE LOWER BACK.

Side-Laying Position

If the receiver prefers to lay on their side during the massage, place pillows between their knees to support the hips and under the top arm for comfort.

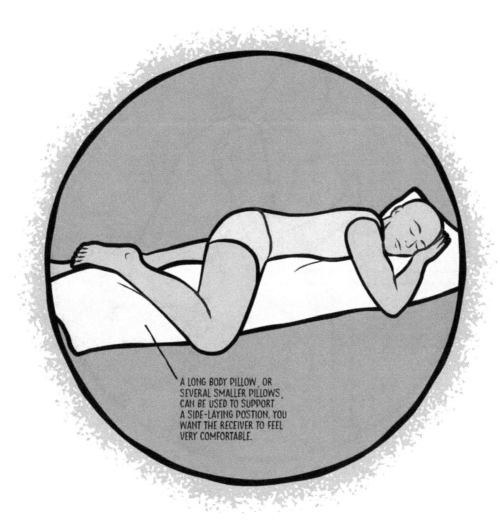

A LONG BODY PILLOW, OR SEVERAL SMALLER PILLOWS, CAN BE USED TO SUPPORT A SIDE-LAYING POSTION. YOU WANT THE RECEIVER TO FEEL VERY COMFORTABLE.

Seated Position

Massage can also be done in a seated position. Give the receiver a pillow to hug as a support when leaning forward on.

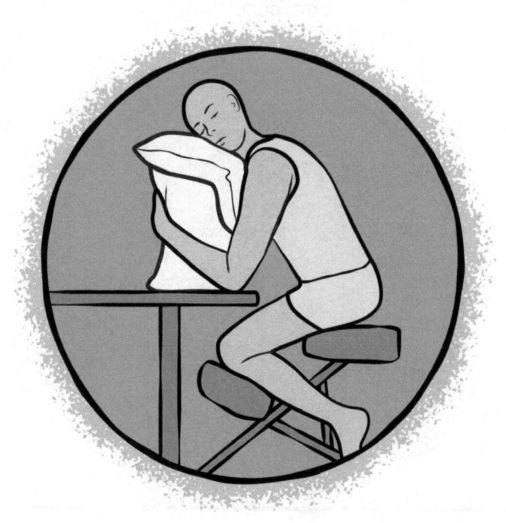

OPENING A SESSION

The way you open a massage session is very important for establishing trust and helping the receiver feel at ease. Make sure you allow time to prepare the space before the receiver arrives (see here).

The massage should be tailored to the receiver's needs, so start by asking what they would like you to focus on and whether they have any specific areas or issues they would like to address. Give them a few moments of privacy to undress and position themselves comfortably, with a towel or sheet covering them. This is a good time to excuse yourself and wash your hands before the session.

Order of Strokes

Start with gentle **compression** strokes through the sheet or towel. You should work rhythmically and slowly, moving with the receiver's breath, sinking in on every exhale and releasing the compression on every inhale. Make sure you are only moving along soft areas of muscle, not pressing on bones or sensitive areas.

Ask the receiver whether they feel warm enough to remove the towel or sheet. Rub a small amount of oil between your palms by moving your hands together until warm. Start with **effleurage** to introduce your touch in long, gliding strokes, working along the length of the area and gliding back slowly. Always open your sessions with lighter pressure that gets slowly deeper, proceeding to kneading **petrissage**, before doing the deeper work of **stripping** or **friction**.

By always using this order of strokes, you will warm up an area properly before working more deeply.

CLOSING A SESSION

Peacefully closing a session is just as important as opening one. The closing routine signals to the receiver that the session is ending, and provides a peaceful space for them to breathe and feel the effects of the lovely work you have been doing.

Finishing Touches

Bring the massage to an end by using long, gliding **effleurage** strokes. These are soothing and calming when done slowly over the length of an area, and are especially nice any time you've done deeper work.

Some quiet energy work can be appropriate. Take the receiver's feet or cradle their head in your hands. Hold still for a few moments, allowing them to breathe and take a peaceful, quiet moment before returning to the world.

Slowly turn on any lights, and keep noise to a minimum. Leave the room to allow the receiver to get dressed.

HAND POSITIONS

During a massage you will use different strokes and therefore different hand positions and actions, working with flat palms, fingers, thumbs, and fingertips, fists, forearms, and elbows.

Flat palms

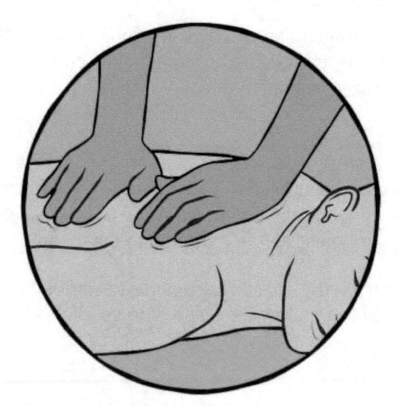

Use a flat palm position for the initial compression work, for spreading oil and warming up an area, and for the gliding effleurage strokes.

Fingers and Thumbs

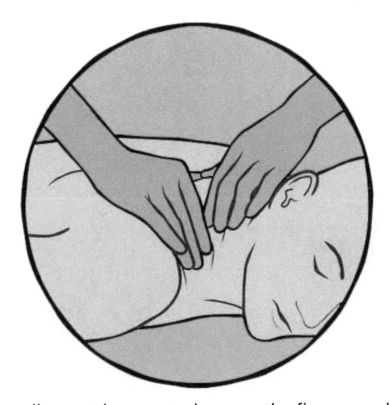

For the kneading petrissage strokes, use the fingers and thumbs to squeeze, wring, and grasp, and lift up muscles.

Hand over Hand

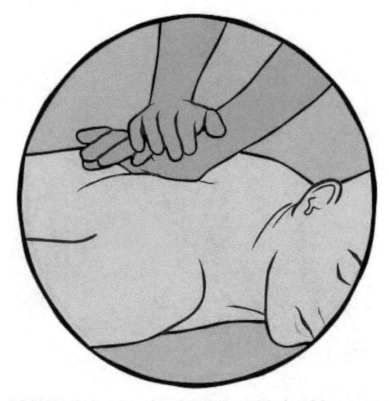

Use one hand over the other for deeper compression strokes, slowly sinking into the muscle with the flat part of your palms and keeping your fingers relaxed. You can also walk one hand next to the other, working across the receiver's body.

Fingertips

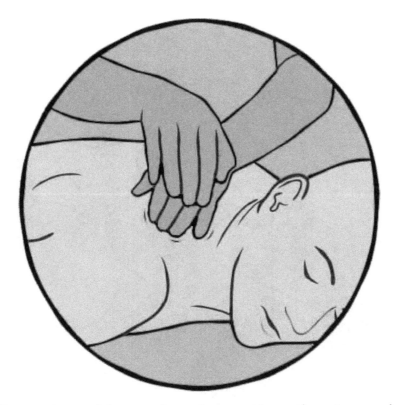

Use your fingertips with one hand over the other to work along the length of the muscles for stripping and cross-fiber friction, and to apply more pressure with a compression stroke.

Relaxed Fist

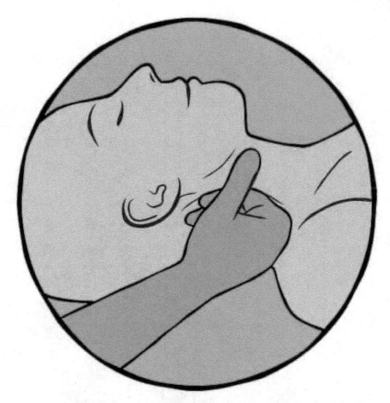

A relaxed fist can be used for rhythmic tapping or tapotement, or for getting into curved areas such as the side of the neck.

Forearm

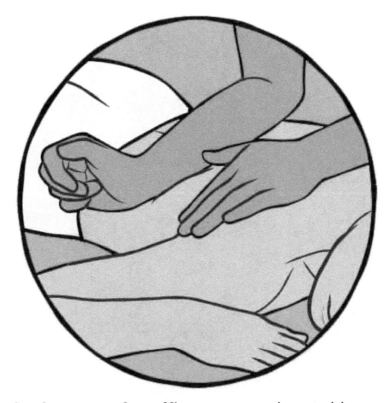

You can use the forearms for effleurage strokes, taking some pressure off the hands, especially on lengthy parts of the body such as along the back or the backs of legs.

Guided Elbow

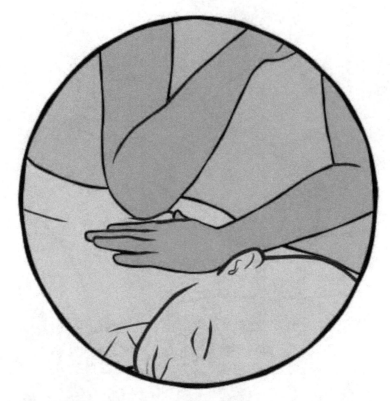

Use a guided elbow position for deep compression work. Make sure to check in about pressure, and work slowly along muscular and fleshy surfaces only, never over bones. Wrap the opposite hand around the base of the elbow for stability.

MASSAGE FOR SHOULDERS

A lot of pain and tension resides in the shoulders, making this area one of the most popular and much-needed for massage.

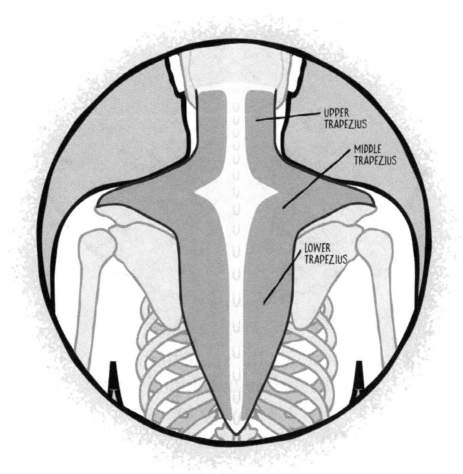

The largest of the shoulder muscle groups is the trapezius group, comprised of upper, middle, and lower sections. The muscle fibers are oriented in many different directions, making them prime areas for adhesions and tension. If the receiver is stressed and their shoulders held up near their ears, a muscle in the trapezius group is most likely to blame.

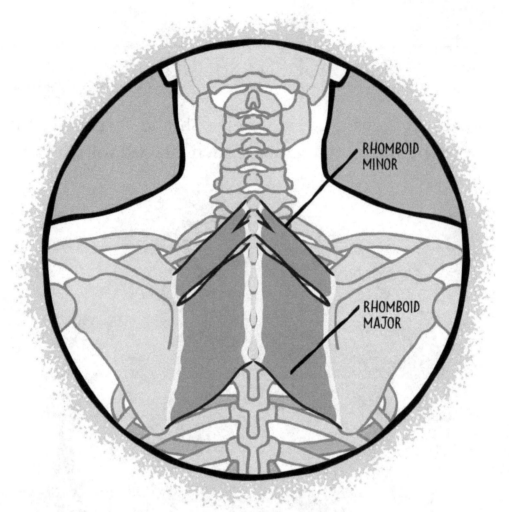

The **rhomboid** muscles attach the spine to the shoulder blade, and are the source of a lot of **tension** and shoulder pain. This muscle group pulls the shoulders back toward the spine, and can feel stiff or achy in people who do a lot of computer work. There are often large **trigger points** found in these muscles, as well as big **adhesions**.

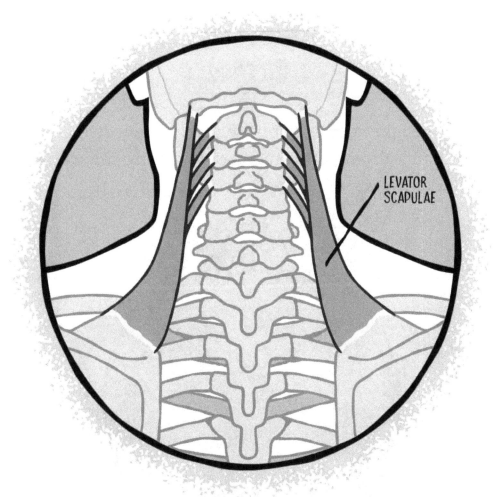

The most commonly complained-about muscle in the shoulder for pain or **tension** is the **levator scapulae**. It attaches the top of the shoulder blade to the neck. When in pain, it feels like a deep and specific ache that travels from the shoulder into the neck.

Method

Position the receiver comfortably laying on their stomach. Start by applying long, gliding effleurage strokes using the palms of the hands to warm up the tissue and spread the oil.

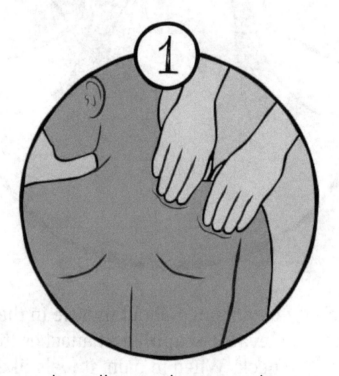

After effleurage, use kneading petrissage strokes to warm up the tops of the shoulders, slowly working the upper trapezius between your hands by picking up the layers of muscles in a slow, repetitive motion and grasping them intermittently between both hands. Use a moderate amount of pressure, focusing on squeezing gently while feeling what's beneath your fingertips.

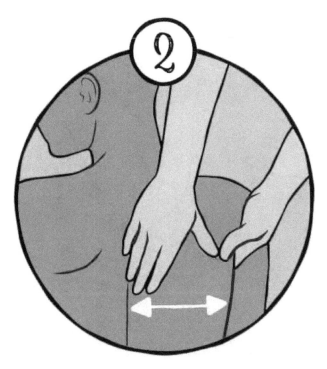

Address the middle trapezius and rhomboids by tracing the length of the muscles with a stripping stroke.

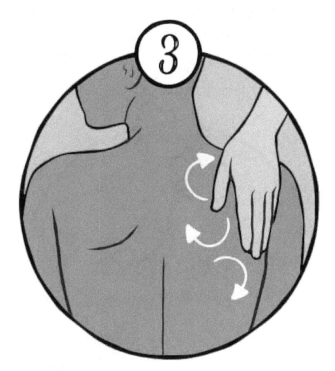

Use a circular friction stroke to work from the top of the shoulders along the length of the shoulder blade, between the spine and levator scapulae, being careful to avoid the bones of the spine. Ask the receiver about the pressure, and be sure to check in regularly.

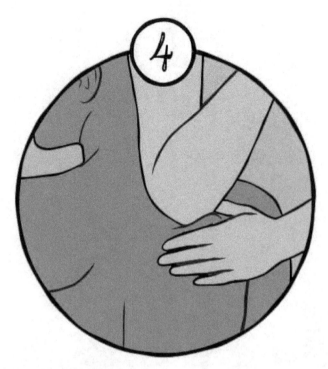

When you notice areas of adhesions, pay special attention. Slow your work down, using a deeper friction stroke to work across layers of muscle and help bring circulation and movement. If cross-fiber friction feels too intense to the receiver, use fingertips or a guided elbow (above) to apply compression to the area.

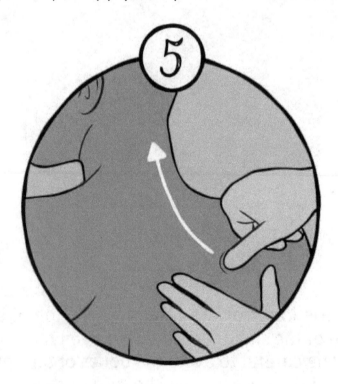

Use your thumb and fingertips to trace along the length of the levator scapulae from the top of the shoulder blade to the neck (above). Use a stripping stroke to feel for any tension, and a cross-fiber stroke to alleviate knots. Use a compression stroke to address trigger points. Close the session with **effleurage** strokes from neck to shoulders to lower back. You can also use these strokes between deeper work to encourage blood flow and soothe any achy areas.

📌
REMINDER

A trigger point feels like a bubble on water. You'll know that you've found a trigger point when the receiver feels a pain-referral pattern. For example, trigger points in levator scapulae can lead to pain or tension in the head and neck.

MASSAGE FOR BACK

The back contains many layers of muscle, running in various directions. Massaging the back is very rewarding, and can be beneficial to anyone experiencing back pain, stiffness, or tension.

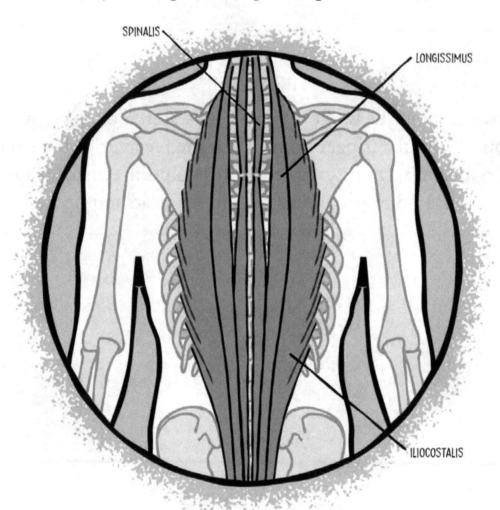

The erector spinae group is a set of three muscles that runs up and down the length of the whole back. Made up of the spinalis, longissimus, and iliocostalis, these muscles help us to stand upright, and can be easily irritated by our daily activities. Erector spinae pain can be felt along the length of the back after a long day on your feet or sitting very still at a desk.

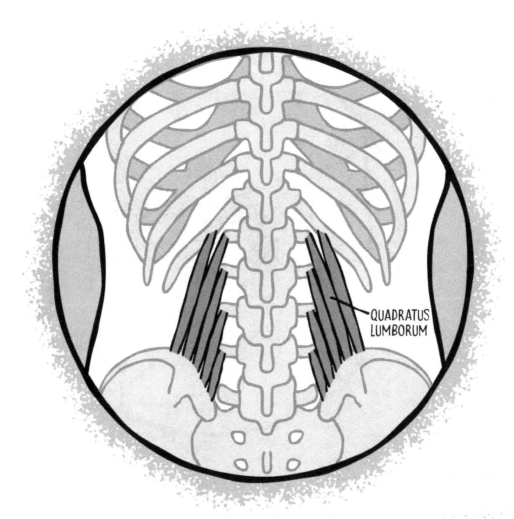

A muscle that commonly impacts lower back pain is **quadratus lumborum**, which attaches the ribs and lower back to the hips. Many **adhesions** are felt where quadratus lumborum layers intersect with the **erector spinae** group. Quadratus lumborum pain feels like a deep ache in the lower back that can radiate down into the sacrum.

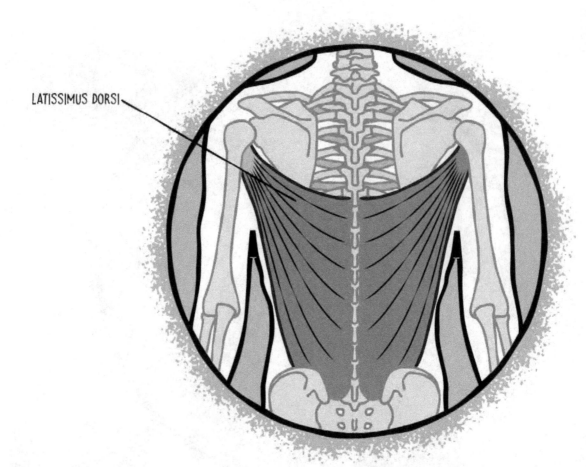

LATISSIMUS DORSI

One of the largest muscles in the back, **latissimus dorsi** helps control movement in the shoulders. When tense, it creates pain that can be felt in the mid- and lower back, and as high up as the shoulders.

Method

Position the receiver comfortably laying on their stomach. Use the flat part of both palms to glide effleurage strokes down the receiver's back to warm the tissues and spread the oil. Travel the full length of the back, from the top of the neck to the very base of the lower back, before returning.

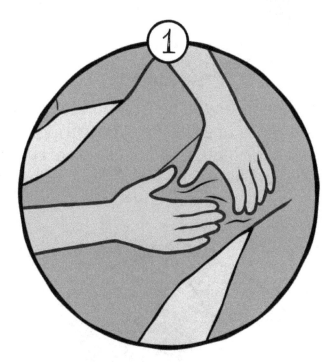

Address each area of the back one at a time. Start with effleurage strokes, then move on to the kneading stroke of petrissage (above) to bring circulation to the area, picking up the layers of muscles and kneading them between your hands.

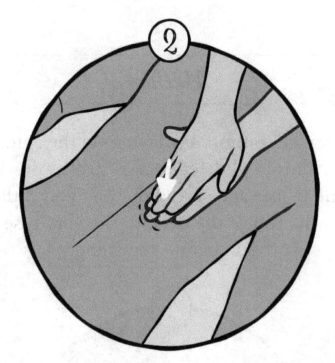

Use a stripping stroke followed by friction along the length of the muscles to address areas of adhesions. For stripping of the erector spinae, place hand over hand (above) for greater depth, applying pressure with your fingers while gliding deeply along the muscles next to the spine.

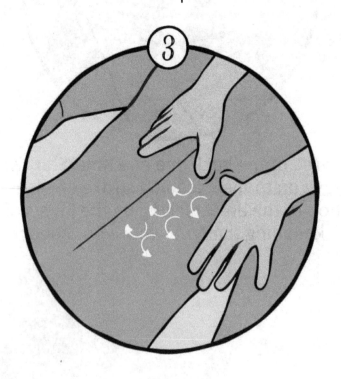

Try using a circular-friction stroke, making small, deep circles along the length of the muscles with your thumbs. Some people may find this stroke a little sensitive in areas of pain, in which case try applying slow and gentle compression, increasing your depth of pressure with the receiver's breathing, to their level of tolerance.

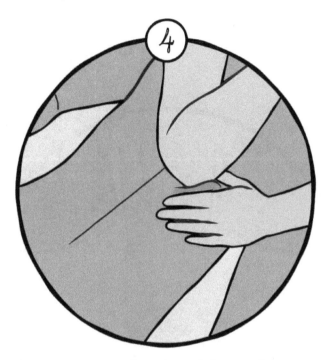

Use a guided elbow to very slowly address the erector spinae and quadratus lumborum muscles. Surround the elbow with the thumb and fingers of the opposite hand to help move it along safely. Firmly sink the guided elbow into the soft, fleshy muscles alongside the spine. There are often trigger points in these areas. Carefully avoid the spine, and make sure to use very slow pressure, regularly checking in with the receiver.

Close the session with **effleurage** strokes from neck to shoulders to lower back. You can also use these strokes between deeper work to encourage blood flow and soothe any achy areas.

MASSAGE FOR NECK

This massage can be especially satisfying and relaxing for anyone who experiences neck tension, headaches, neck stiffness from daily activities, or strain from using a computer or cell phone.

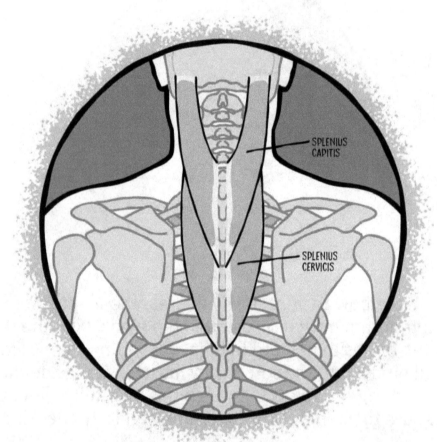

Splenius capitis and splenius cervicis connect the upper back and neck to the base of the head, and help the head to stay in an upright position. Pain or tension in these muscles can be felt along the neck and into the head.

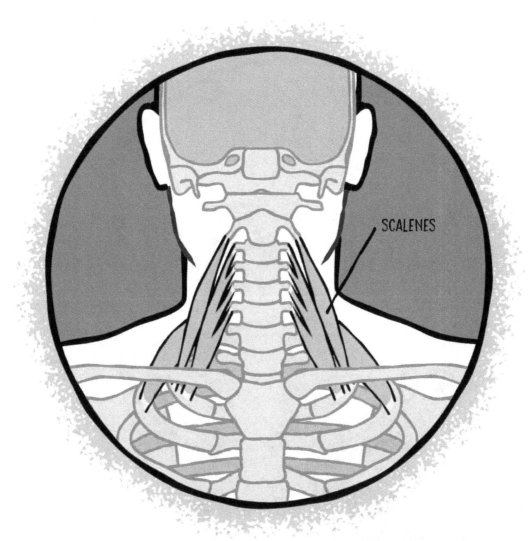

The **scalenes** attach the neck to the ribs and shoulders, and act by bending the neck to the same side, as well as helping to elevate the upper ribs on a deep breath. Spasms felt in the scalenes can refer pain all the way from the neck down into the arm and even the chest, as well as the side of the head. **Trigger points** in scalenes can cause bad headaches.

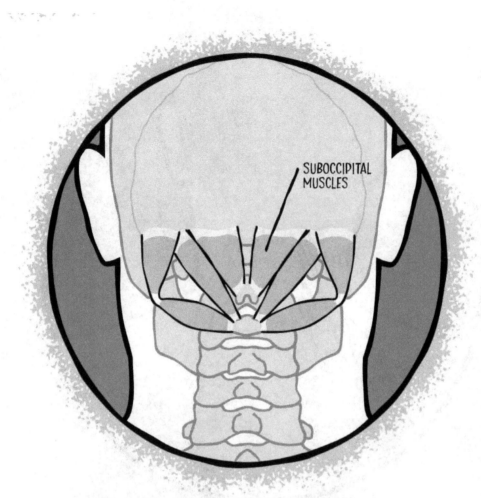

The **suboccipital** muscles attach the base of the skull to the top of the spine, and are reflexively linked to vision. **Tension** or spasms in this group cause headaches that can be felt all along the sides of the head and temples. **Trigger points** in the suboccipitals can also cause migraine headaches.

Method

Position the receiver comfortably laying face down or seated. For the initial effleurage strokes, use the flat part of both your palms to glide the oil slowly down the receiver's neck, from the base of the skull to the tops of the shoulders and back.

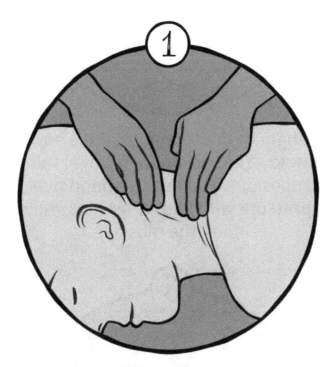

Address each area of the neck one at a time. Start with effleurage strokes, then, for petrissage, use a pickup kneading stroke along the length of the fleshy part of the back of the neck, paying attention to any areas that feel tense. You can also pick up on tension in some of the scalene muscles by focusing gently on the sides of the neck.

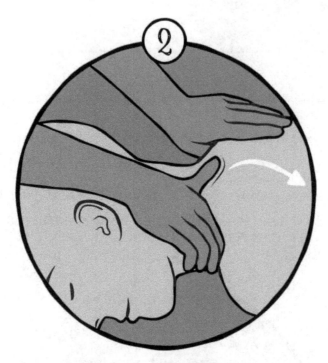

Work along the length of the splenius capitis and splenius cervicis muscles using a muscle stripping stroke (above) followed by friction to address areas of adhesions. You can use hand over hand for greater depth, applying pressure with your fingertips while gliding deeply along the muscles.

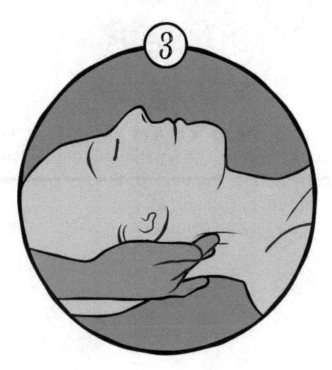

To more deeply address the scalenes and suboccipitals, position the receiver on their back and follow the steps of effleurage, petrissage, stripping, and circular or cross-fiber friction to address tension. Check in with the receiver on the pressure and adjust as necessary.

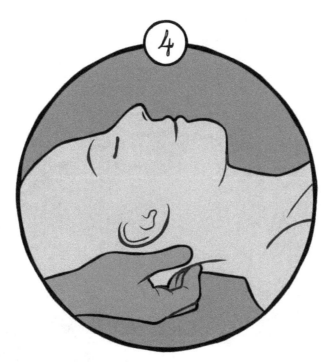

To release the suboccipital muscles, use a scooping motion under the receiver's neck to slowly bring your fingers toward the base of their skull. Press up toward the ceiling and hold this spot while the receiver breathes deeply in and out. You'll feel the muscles start to soften and release. Be sure to check in with the receiver about the pressure.

To close the neck session, use lots of gentle **petrissage** strokes with light to medium pressure. Follow with slow and sweeping **effleurage** strokes to close the session and encourage circulation.

MASSAGE FOR ARMS

Massaging the upper and lower arms is useful for injury prevention from typing, or any repetitive movement, ranging from carrying groceries to lifting up a child.

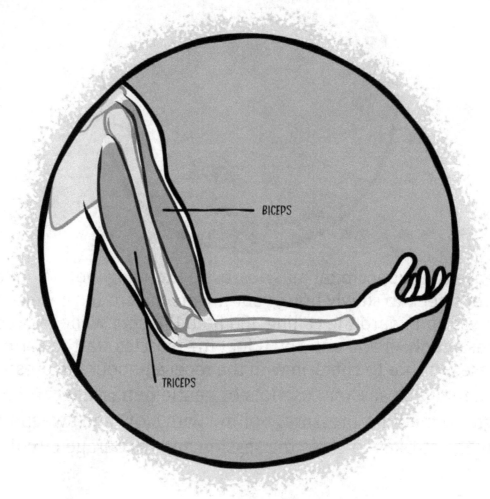

The major muscles in the upper arms include the biceps muscle, which bends the arm, and the triceps, which acts to straighten it.

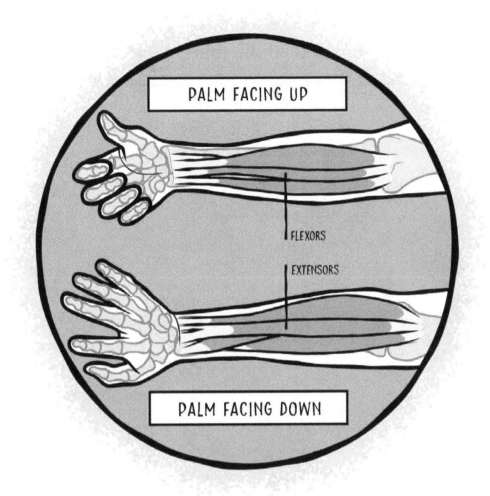

In the lower arm we have **flexor** muscles on the palm side of the wrist and forearm that curl the hand toward us, and **extensor** muscles on the other side that pull the hand back.

Flexors: If you look at the palm of your hand, cup it, and bring it toward you, you are using the flexors.

Extensors: If you hold your arm with the palm facing down and bring your hand toward you, you are using the extensors.

DANGER ZONE

Be cautious at the sensitive part of the elbow where the ulnar nerve (sometimes called the funny bone) is exposed.

Method

Position the receiver comfortably laying on their back. For the warming effleurage strokes, use the flat part of both palms to glide the oil slowly from the base of the receiver's wrist to the top of their arm, over their shoulder, and back down to the hand.

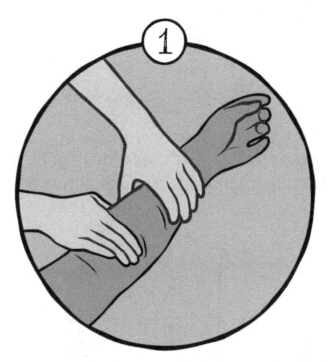

After effleurage, use a kneading petrissage stroke to bring circulation to the area, picking up the layers of muscles and kneading them between your hands, paying attention to any spots that are tense. Be careful to avoid the sensitive area at the elbow.

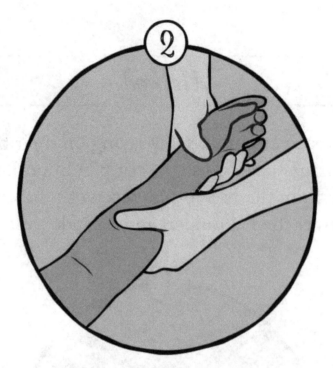

When the muscles are thoroughly warmed up, follow along their length using a muscle stripping stroke from wrist to elbow followed by friction to address areas of adhesions.

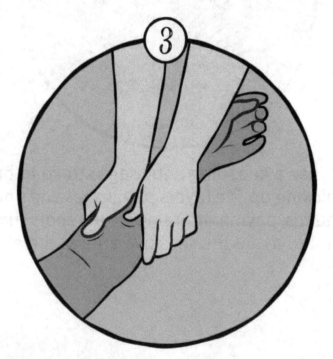

For muscle stripping of the biceps, extensors, and flexors, place hand over hand for greater depth, applying pressure with your fingertips while gliding deeply along the muscles. You can also circle the arm with your hands and gently squeeze while moving from wrist to elbow, as though squeezing a tube of toothpaste.

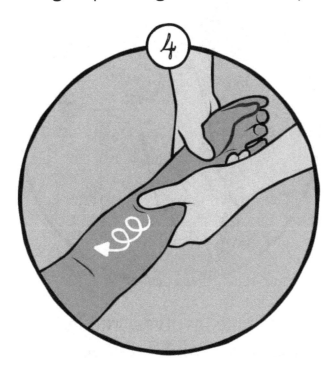

Apply cross-fiber friction along the length of the arm, gliding your fingers across the muscles and moving slowly back and forth from the outside of the arm to the inside. You can also use a circular friction stroke (above), making small, deep circles along the length of the muscles with your thumbs. Start with the palm face up to address the flexor muscles, then gently turn the palm over to work on the extensor muscles.

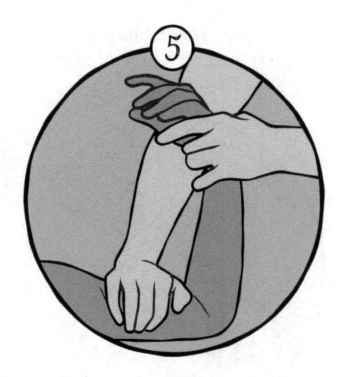

Another enjoyable technique involves "ruddering" the arm. Bend the arm at the elbow and gently hold the receiver's hand, guiding the arm back and forth as you apply pressure to the **biceps** muscle. This is a nice passive way to work on the muscle.

Close the session with **effleurage** strokes from the fingertips toward the top of the arm. You can also use these strokes between deeper work to encourage blood flow and soothe any achy areas.

MASSAGE FOR HANDS

Hand massage is wonderfully relaxing, and can be carried out in any setting with ease. Be careful to use milder pressure, since hands can be especially sensitive.

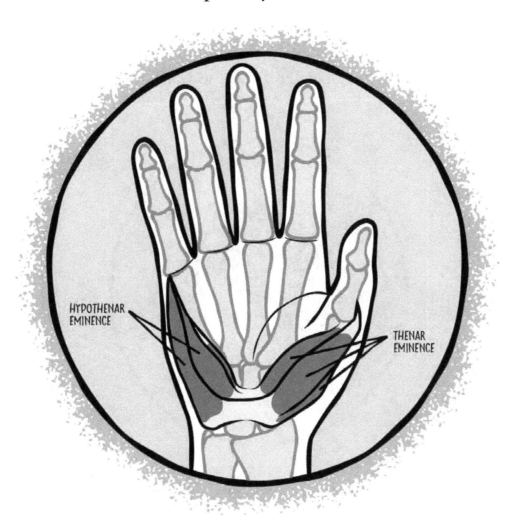

The fleshy part of the palm by the base of the thumb is called the thenar eminence. The fleshy part of the palm by the base of the little finger is the hypothenar eminence. These are both great places to focus on in a hand massage.

Method

Position the receiver comfortably, either seated or laying face up, and hold their hand in both of yours. Use the flat part of both thumbs to make slow, gliding effleurage strokes from the center of the palm moving out toward the fingertips in a fanning motion. Work your way through all of the fingers. This also provides a gentle stretch to the hand.

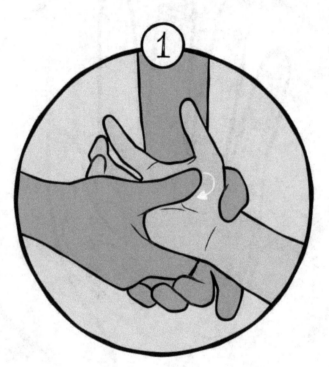

For the kneading stroke of petrissage, focus on the thenar eminence, pinching it gently between your thumb and forefinger and applying pressure in a circular motion. You'll likely find a lot of tension here.

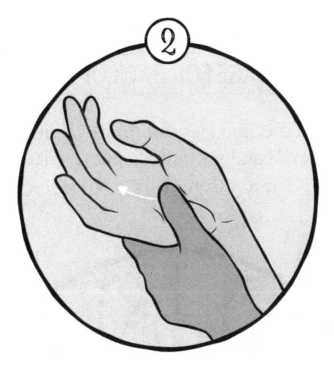

Work gently on each finger separately, being careful not to pull too hard. Check in with the receiver on the pressure. Use stripping strokes to work your way around the palm from the thenar eminence to the hypothenar eminence.

Close the session with more relaxing **effleurage** strokes.

MASSAGE FOR BACK OF LEGS

Massaging the backs of the legs can improve circulation, help the legs feel more relaxed and grounded, and alleviate any soreness or tension from daily activities.

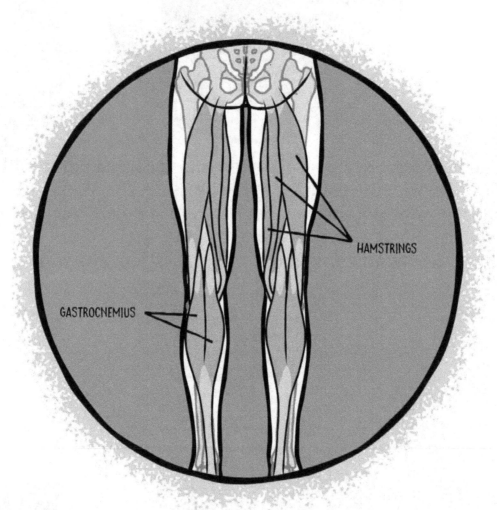

The backs of the legs contain large and lengthy muscles, including the hamstrings on the thighs and the gastrocnemius muscles of the calf.

DANGER ZONE

Be careful when working over the back of the knee, which is a vulnerable soft spot that should only be addressed using light touch. Also be mindful if the receiver has varicose veins, which should be avoided.

Method

Position the receiver comfortably on their stomach with a pillow or rolled towel under their ankles. For the warming effleurage strokes, use the flat part of both palms to glide the oil slowly from the ankle to the hip.

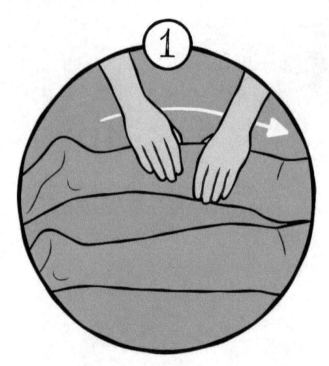

After effleurage, use a pettrisage stroke from ankle to hip, slowly working your way up the leg with both hands to knead the large muscles of the calf, up through the large muscles of the back of the thigh, and return back to the ankle with a long, gliding stroke.

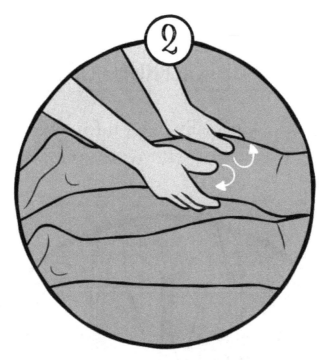

Use your thumbs to apply slow, steady, deeper pressure using a small circular motion from the ankle up to the base of the back of the knee. Spend time on any areas of tension, working with a friction stroke across the muscle with your fingertips.

Close the session with long, relaxing **effleurage** strokes.

STRETCHING TIP

Clasp the receiver's ankle with both hands and lift until the knee is bent, then apply pressure to the top of the foot with one hand and guide the foot toward the buttock. Use a slow, gentle movement—it shouldn't feel forced—and hold this position for two breaths. Relax the leg back down.

MASSAGE FOR FRONT OF LEGS

Leg massage can be especially helpful for anyone who sits for lengthy periods, or who works on their feet.

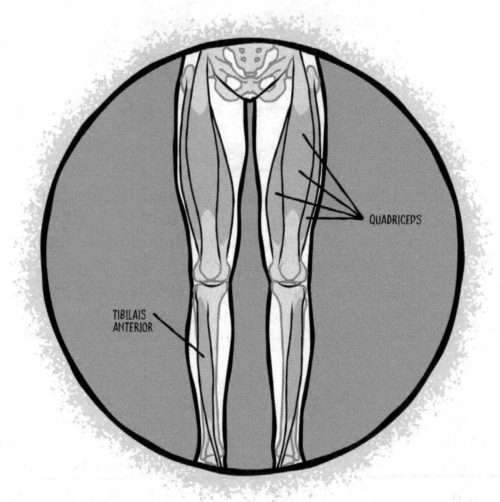

The fronts of the legs have more bony surfaces than the backs of the legs, so a slightly different approach is used on the lower leg. The upper thigh contains the large quadriceps muscles, which are often tense and can handle firm pressure. The lower leg contains the tibilais anterior muscle, which can feel sore from standing and daily movement.

Method

Position the receiver comfortably on their back. Warming the oil between your palms, use effleurage strokes, from ankle to hip, to introduce your touch and spread the oil.

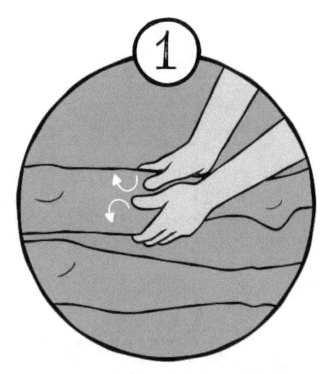

Using your thumbs, follow along the outside edge of the shin from ankle to knee, with small, slow circles, feeling for any areas of tension.

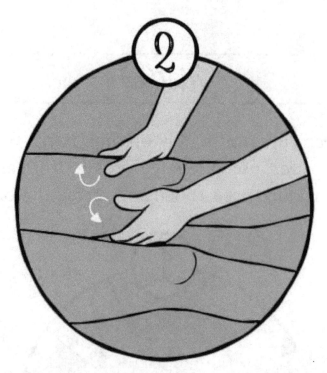

Follow with a petrissage stroke from above the knee to the hip, slowly working your way up the thigh with both hands to knead the muscles. Use open palms and upward circular movements with your thumbs, and return back to the ankle with a long, gliding effleurage stroke.

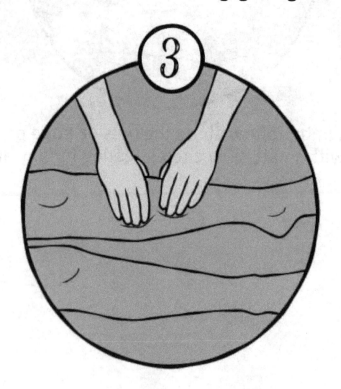

If you feel any areas of tension, spend extra time there, working across the muscle with your fingertips using a friction stroke. Check in with the receiver on the pressure, using compression to achieve more depth if needed.

Close the session with long, gliding **effleurage** stokes.

MASSAGE FOR FEET

Foot massage is extremely popular, and can be helpful for anyone who stands on their feet for lengthy periods, or who wears uncomfortable shoes on a regular basis.

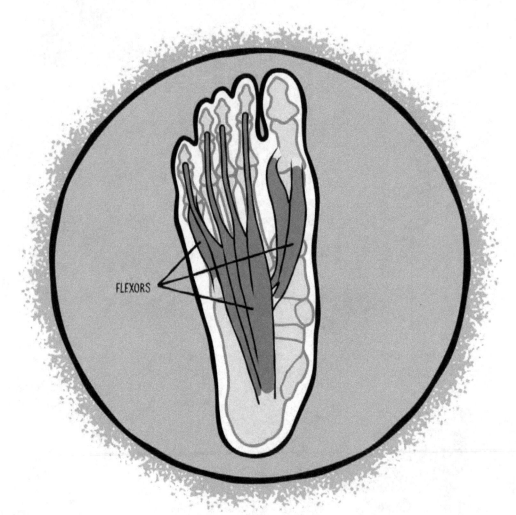

FLEXORS

Foot massage focuses on two opposing muscle groups: flexor muscles on the bottom of the foot, which act to point the toes downward, and extensor muscles on the top of the foot, which point the toes upward.

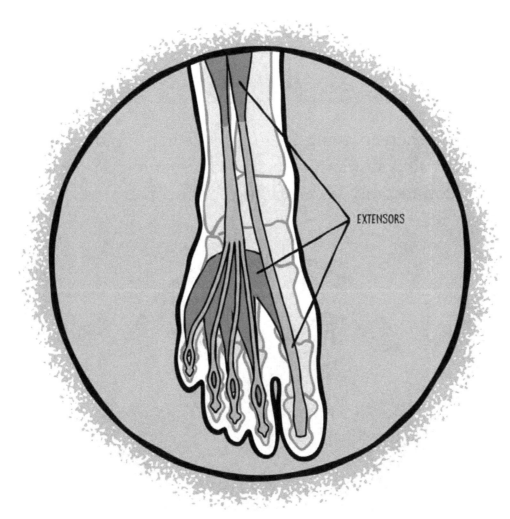

EXTENSORS

TIP

The skin of the feet can be very dry, so choose a thicker
massage cream or foot balm for extra moisturizing properties.

Method

Position the receiver laying face up or sitting. Cradle one foot in both hands, palms holding just next to the ankles. You should be comfortably seated facing the receiver's feet.

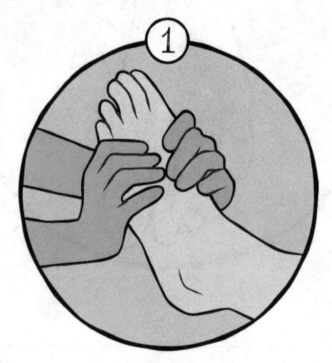

Use a circular motion to start to warm up the ankles and feet, moving the hands at first simultaneously (above) to create some circulation, then altering one after the other to bring the foot into some motion from left to right. To address the heel of the foot, cup the base of the ankle to gently raise the foot, and use the other hand, pressing the thumb into the side of the heel. Work along the length of the heel from one side to the other, making small circles with your thumb.

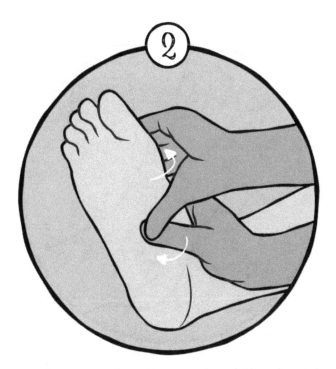

Use a petrissage stroke to wring the arch of the foot by grasping it with both hands and gently twisting the arch in opposite directions with each hand.

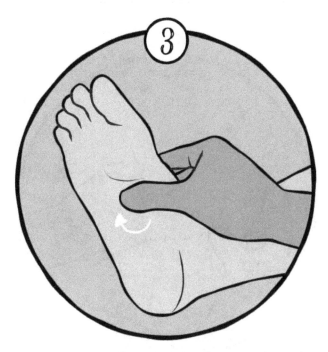

Use your thumb to make a circular friction stroke along the arch of the foot from the heel toward the base of the big toe, checking in regarding pressure.

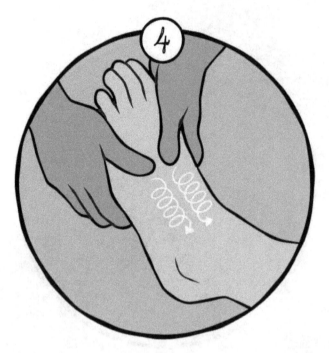

Address the top of the foot and ankle by using warming effleurage and kneading petrissage strokes to make rhythmic movements using your thumbs in slow circles (above), fanning out over the top of the foot from the center to the outsides.

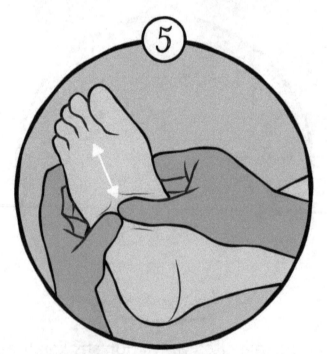

Use a **stripping** stroke to trace the **flexor** muscles by applying pressure from the toes toward the ankle and back again.

Close the session with **effleurage** strokes over the length of the whole foot, and end with a gentle pull on each toe.

MASSAGE FOR HEAD AND SCALP

A head and scalp massage is a relaxing treatment for anyone suffering from headaches or overall stress and tension. Remember to massage very slowly, in time with the receiver's breathing, to keep a relaxing pace.

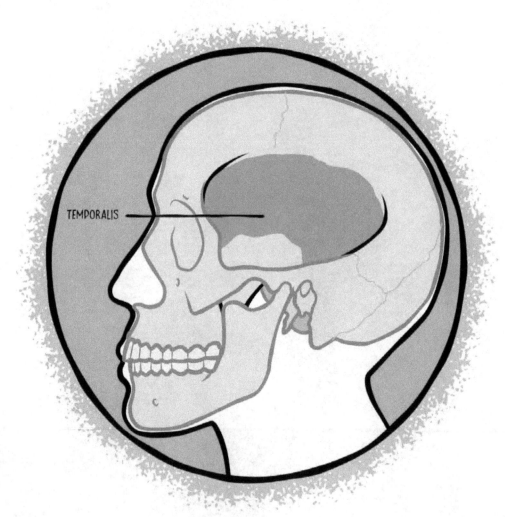

TEMPORALIS

There are many muscular attachments at the base of the head and along the sides, and many nerve endings on the scalp. The temporalis muscle is at the side of the skull.

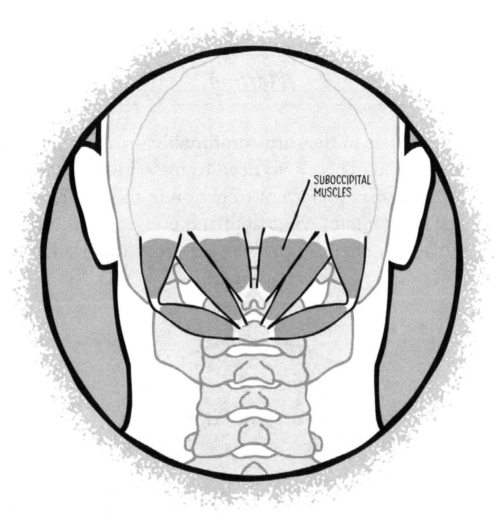

SUBOCCIPITAL
MUSCLES

The suboccipital muscles attach the base of the skull to the top of the
neck. This set of muscles is reflexively linked to vision and often the
cause of tension headaches.

Method

Position the receiver so they are comfortably seated or facing up in a supported position. There's no need to use oil for a head massage, and many people may prefer not to get oil in their hair, so be sure to check first. Be mindful when applying pressure not to tug at the hair, and also to check in on pressure, since the head is very sensitive.

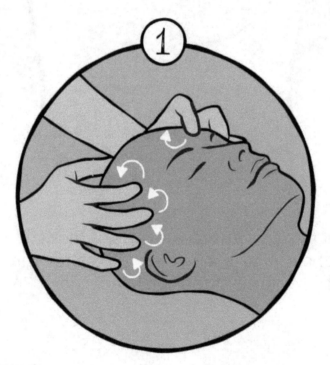

Plant your fingertips firmly on the receiver's head and move in slow, repetitive circles, as though shampooing the hair, to bring circulation to the area and warm it up. Make sure to address the whole head by working underneath and along the sides and front. The slower you work, the more relaxing it will feel.

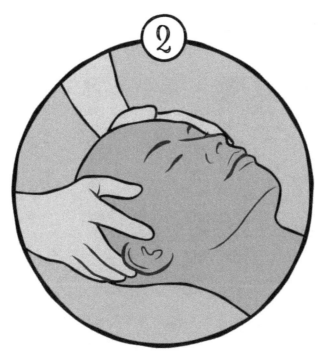

Move your hands to the sides of the temples, placing your fingers above and below the ears in a scissoring movement, to glide down in front of and behind the ears, which have many nerve endings.

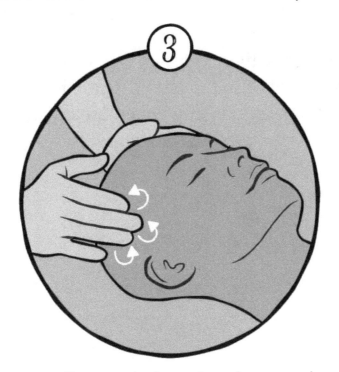

Focus on the temporalis muscle by using slow, moderately pressured circles with both your hands. You can turn the head to one side to focus on the other side.

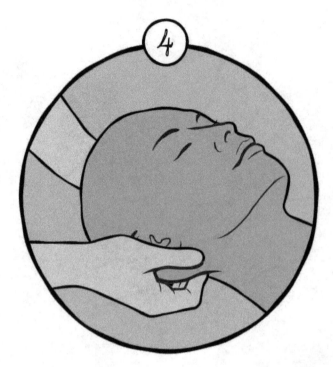

Address the muscles at the base of the skull by applying pressure in slow, steady circles along the top of the neck. You can also use a gentle squeezing motion at the back of the neck to apply pressure to the points on the base of the head. There are often trigger points found in these areas.

Close the massage with increasingly slower circles, using both thumbs to press gently into the crown of the head or the top of the forehead and taking several slow, deep breaths while letting your fingers rest.

MASSAGE FOR FACE

Facial massage can address jaw tension, headaches, and pain due to sinus issues or congestion. It can also help to keep the skin moisturized and bring fresh circulation to the surface, creating a more youthful appearance. The receiver may prefer not to use oil on the face, or you might ask them to provide their favorite non-oily moisturizer or skin serum. Use a small amount only.

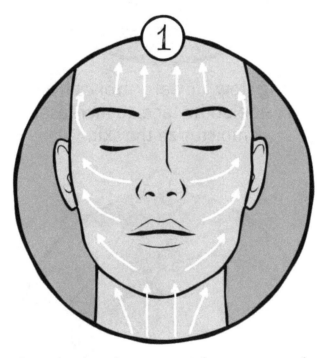

Position the receiver laying face up. When massaging the face, keep strokes facing in an upward motion, toward the top of the head.

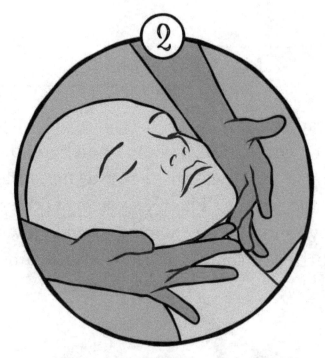

Warm the face by using slow, upward strokes from the neck and light strokes along the side of the face, to increase circulation and moisturize the skin.

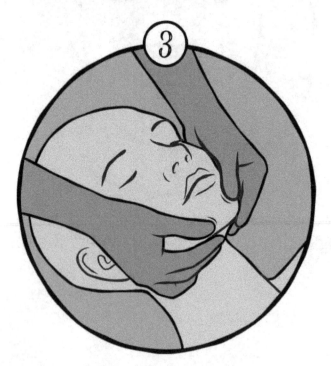

Address the muscles along the jaw with upward, circular strokes to alleviate jaw tension. Notice any areas of adhesion and use compression to address them.

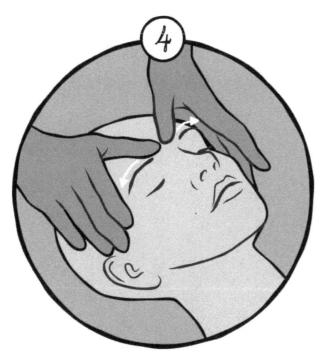

Address the muscles of the forehead with slow compression strokes along the ridge of the eyebrows. Be careful not to tug on the skin.

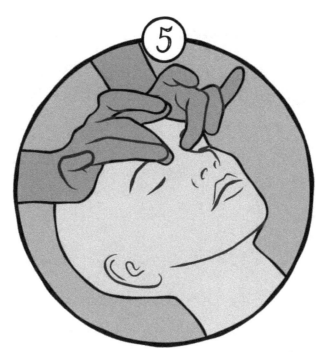

Apply gentle pressure to the points just next to the nose, avoiding the delicate eye area.

To close a facial massage, cup your receiver's ears by hovering your hands just over them. This gives a lovely, warm moment of peace and quiet before you move on to the next area.

MASSAGE FOR RELAXATION

The goal of a relaxation massage is to soothe overtired nerves and calm the full nervous system with very slow, long strokes. Set the mood for your relaxation session by adjusting the light to be very low, perhaps using lavender-scented candles. A low fan can provide some white noise for the background, or you might choose some soft music. Have the receiver lay comfortably face down, with a cushion or pillow under their knees. Stand at their head, facing their body. A massage for relaxation requires only effleurage, the very long, gliding, relaxing strokes.

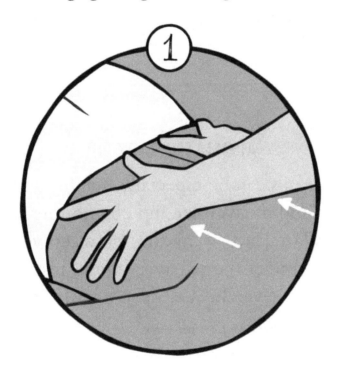

Using a long, sliding effleurage stroke, glide both flat palms down the full length of the receiver's back.

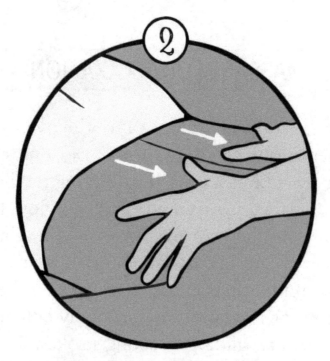

With the returning stroke, use your full forearms and relaxed palms to slowly bring your hands back toward their neck.

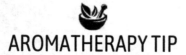

AROMATHERAPY TIP

Using essential oils can be especially helpful with relaxation. Try adding a blend of lavender and chamomile essential oils to your base oil. Warm the oil mixture between your palms, then hold your hands under the receiver's nose, instructing them to take several even, deep breaths in.

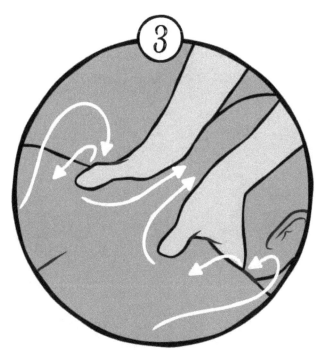

Scoop your arms under the shoulders at the side, then slide up from the top of the shoulders to the base of the neck. This motion should create a diamond shape. Use this stroke pattern on the back, neck, and shoulders, followed by the legs and feet at a slow and steady pace.

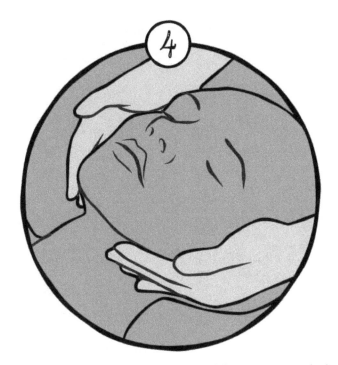

Ask the receiver to turn over, and, working toward the heart, apply effleurage strokes to their feet, legs, arms, shoulders, and neck,

finishing the session with their head and scalp.
Close the session with a slow, deep pause at the temples or the
crown of the head.

5 TREATMENT PLANS

Each of us has a unique part to play in the healing of the world.

MARIANNE WILLIAMSON

MASSAGE FOR HEADACHES

Headaches can be caused by tension, migraines, anxiety, allergies, and stress. Some headaches are felt at the base of the head or along the temples, while others feel like pressure or sharp pain. Regardless of their cause, massage is a very effective way of helping treat a headache by applying pressure to specific areas that are known to reduce pain.

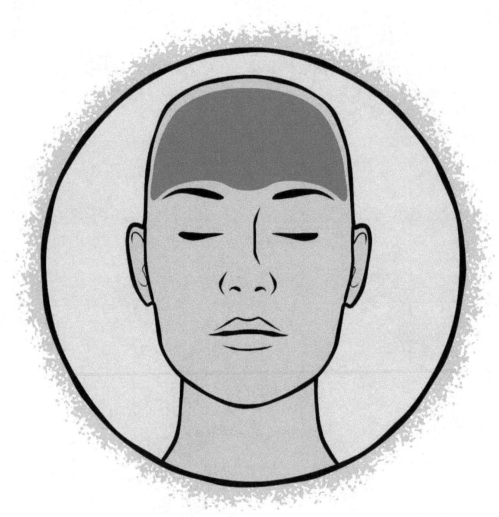

!
WORD OF CAUTION

Massage for a headache caused by a fever should be avoided until the receiver is feeling better.

AROMATHERAPY TIP

Try adding a few drops of peppermint essential oil to a base oil and gently massage this into the base of the neck. Do not use peppermint oil straight, as this can be irritating to some people. Avoid using peppermint oil directly on the face, since it might irritate the eyes.

Method

To treat a headache, work very slowly and deliberately, and follow the protocol to warm up the muscles of the neck and shoulders using long, gliding effleurage strokes and kneading petrissage strokes.

When the receiver is feeling relaxed and warm, apply pressure using the pace of several slow, deep breaths, to the areas illustrated, which may be tender.

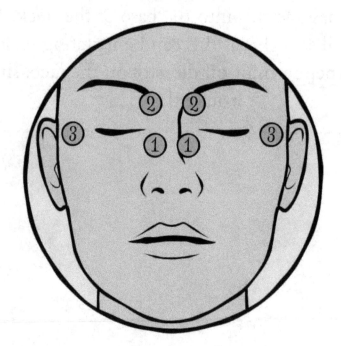

1) Below the inner corner of the eyes.

2) Just above point 1, pressing upward.

3) Along the temples.

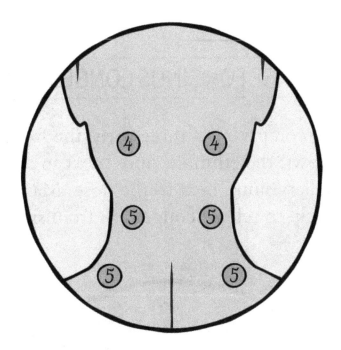

④ At the base of the skull.

⑤ At the **levator scapulae**, which can refer pain up into the head.

MASSAGE FOR SINUS CONGESTION

The sinuses are comprised of three parts: the frontal sinus, just above the eyebrows; the ethmoid sinus, next to the corner of the eye; and the maxillary sinus, next to the nose. Massaging these areas will help to release congestion from sinuses.

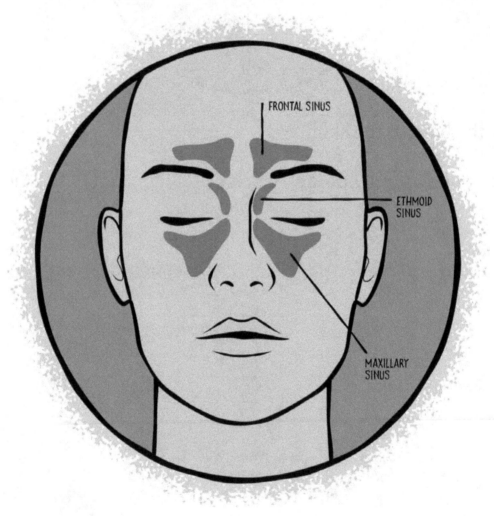

Method

Treating sinus pain or congestion with massage involves applying pressure to particular areas of the face.

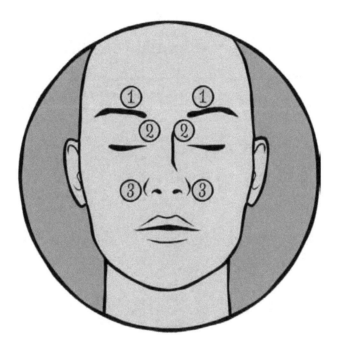

(1) Just above the eyebrows using a light upward and inward motion.

(2) Between the eyes and the corners of the nose, using a light upward and inward motion.

(3) Lastly, apply pressure to the base of the nose, just next to where the nostrils meet the face. Make sure to check in with the receiver about the amount of pressure being applied.

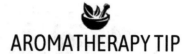

AROMATHERAPY TIP

For additional benefit, a combination of eucalyptus and rosemary essential oils can be blended into a base oil and applied to the chest, or inhaled with steam or on a warm washcloth. Avoid aromatherapy use around the eyes, since this can be irritating. Do not apply essential oils directly to the skin.

MASSAGE FOR CONSTIPATION

Constipation occurs when bowel movements are infrequent or hard to pass, and can happen due to a lack of fiber in the diet, or because of certain medications. Abdominal massage can be extremely helpful in relieving this condition.

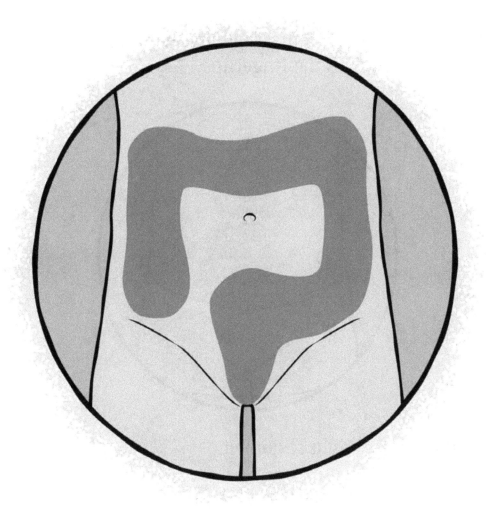

Method

The small intestine flows into the colon, traveling up the right side of the body (ascending colon), across the midsection (transverse colon), before turning down toward the rectum (descending colon). Your massage should follow the path of the colon.

The protocol for abdominal massage involves applying slow, small, gentle circle strokes with the fingertips.

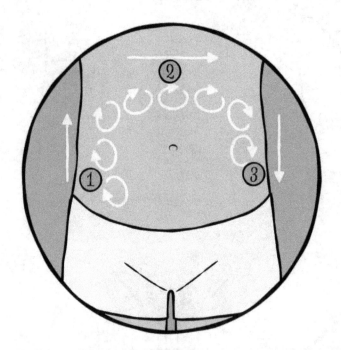

(1) Start at the lower right abdomen.

(2) Travel across the midsection.

(3) Continue down the left side of the abdomen, along the route of the colon. Use moderate to lighter pressure depending on the receiver's level of comfort.

!

WORD OF CAUTION

Abdominal massage is not appropriate for anyone who is pregnant, or those suffering from high blood pressure or a heart condition.

MASSAGE FOR MENSTRUAL CRAMPS

Menstrual cramps are caused by contractions of the uterine muscle, which can create pain in the abdomen and lower back.

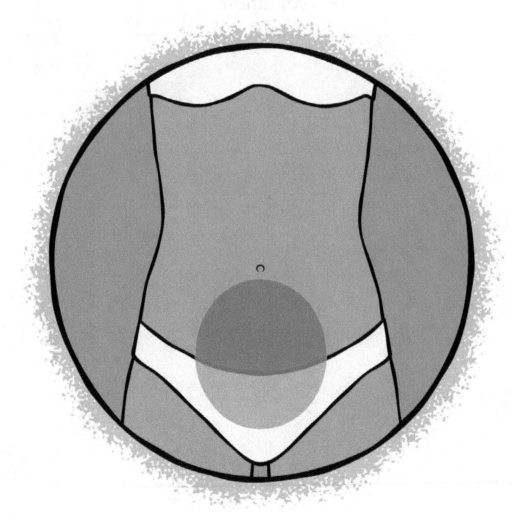

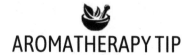

AROMATHERAPY TIP

For added benefit, blend essential oil of rose geranium, known in Ayurvedic medicine for its hormone-balancing properties, with your base massage oil.

Method

For stress relief, focus a massage on the neck, shoulders, and deep lower back (see here), using slow compression holds over areas of pain or tension. Check in with the receiver and work within their level of tolerance.

Start by applying a heat pack to the lower back or abdomen to reduce cramps.

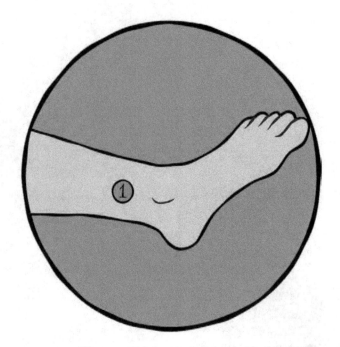

1. After applying a stress-relieving neck, shoulder, and back massage, apply pressure for six to ten seconds to the acupressure point on the ankle (pictured).

2. Apply pressure for six to ten seconds to the acupressure point on the abdomen (pictured) to help alleviate cramping.

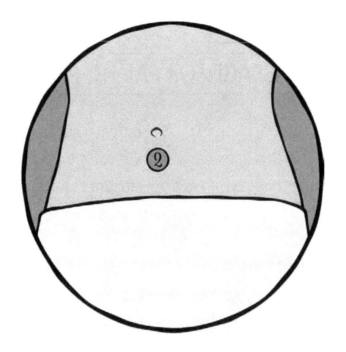

TIP

Following the session, give the receiver a cup of organic raspberry leaf tea for extra menstrual support.

MASSAGE FOR PAIN RELIEF

To relieve pain caused by muscle tension or trigger points, long, steady compression holds can be very effective. Always make sure to check in with the receiver on the pressure and look for other physical or visual cues of discomfort or pain, such as a grimace, tensing up a body part, or holding their breath. Ask the receiver for feedback on a scale of one to ten, with one being too light and ten being too painful. You should aim for a six or seven, and asking for specific numbers can help you to adjust accordingly.

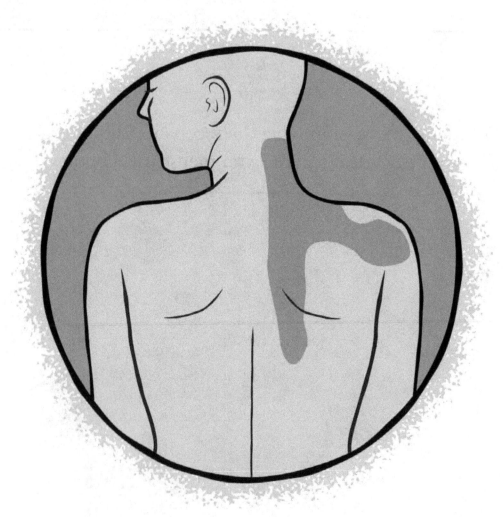

Method

For a pain-relieving session, work slowly and specifically, using anatomy to guide you. Start the massage by asking the receiver what specifically is hurting them, and when you begin to work on an area, ask them if they'd prefer pressure "higher up, lower down, to the left, or right" and subtly adjust until you are in the right location.

A pain-relieving session may not be a full-body approach; sometimes the receiver will just want you to focus on the painful area. Warm the area with **effleurage** and **petrissage** before using deeper **stripping** or **cross-fiber friction** work.

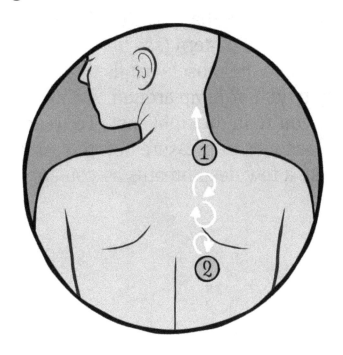

!
WORD OF CAUTION

For pain caused by illness or injury, massage therapy is not indicated.

1. After **effleurage** and **petrissage**, use **stripping** strokes along the length of the muscle.

2. Use **cross-fiber friction** across the belly of the muscle. Friction can feel very intense for some, in which case use a **compression** stroke to apply moderate to deep pressure to the area, slowly increasing it with their breath and tolerance. Remember to avoid working directly over areas of bones, bruises, or injury.

3. A **trigger point** feels to the touch like a bubble on water, and the receiver will remark that pressing the point feels good and creates a pain-referral pattern (see here). You may also notice a "jump sign," where the muscle bands that you are compressing start to subtly twitch or jump around. A jump sign is a strong indicator that you're in the right spot. To treat a trigger point, use six to ten seconds of pressure before easing off. Ask the receiver to take a few deep breaths as you apply pressure.

MASSAGE FOR INSOMNIA

Insomnia is regular sleeplessness, or the inability to sleep, and is often caused by stress or anxiety. Research has shown that regular massage increases the receiver's ability to relax, and can help restore healthy sleep patterns.

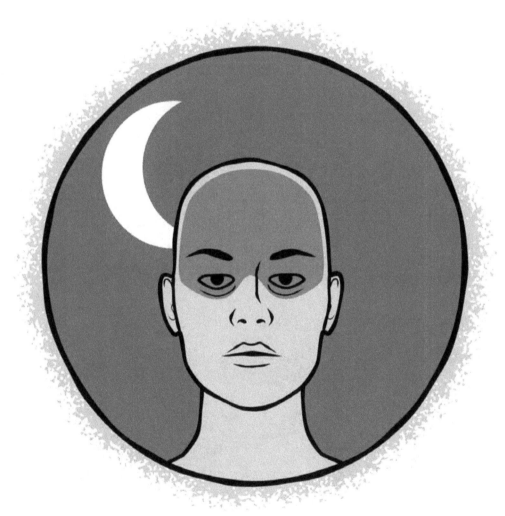

Method

Massage to help with sleep starts with very repetitive, slow effleurage strokes anywhere on the body. The key is that the strokes should become slightly slower with each pass. Encourage the receiver to synchronize a deep breath in with the rhythm of your movement.

A very slow, rhythmic scalp massage can be especially helpful (see here).

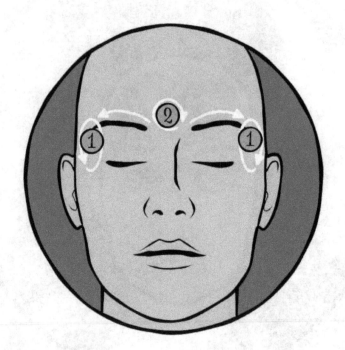

① Use your middle fingers to make slow circles at the temples.

② Use your middle fingers to make slow circles between the eyebrows, then trace over the curve of the eyebrows.

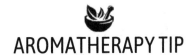

AROMATHERAPY TIP

Add a combination of lavender and chamomile essential oils to the base oil to help the receiver to relax before bed. This blend can also be added to a bath before bed, or sprayed onto a pillow for continued nighttime use.

MASSAGE FOR INFLAMMATION

Massage is only helpful in cases of chronic inflammation (see here). In the case of acute or recent inflammation, when there's been a new injury or new swelling that is unusual, avoid putting any pressure on the area: instead use ice, elevate the area, and encourage rest or medical attention when needed. In the case of chronic or longer-term inflammation, very light massage can be helpful in bringing circulation to the area.

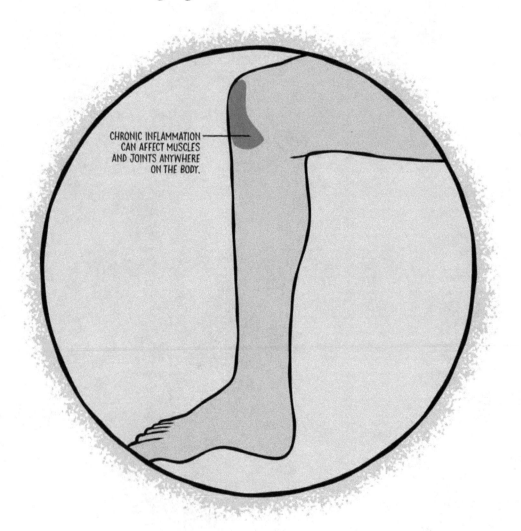

CHRONIC INFLAMMATION CAN AFFECT MUSCLES AND JOINTS ANYWHERE ON THE BODY.

Method

The special type of work that can be done on an area of chronic inflammation is called lymphatic drainage massage, because it affects the lymphatic fluid responsible for causing the swelling. This type of massage is extremely light and rhythmic, and works to slowly help reduce inflammation in the area by encouraging the lymphatic fluid to drain in the direction of the nearest lymph nodes.

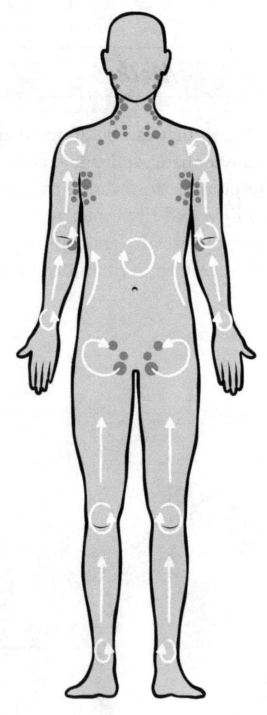

① Lymph nodes are found in the areas shown. Begin at the
farthest area affected by the inflammation, working toward the
local lymph node and moving in the direction of the heart.

(2) Apply pressure light enough to only just move the surface of the skin, in a slow and steady, sweeping rhythm.

(3) Travel in the direction of the heart to the nearest lymph node—for example, from toes to foot to knee to hip, or from fingers to hands to elbows to upper arms. Check in regularly with the receiver—this should not feel painful.

!

WORD OF CAUTION

Do not massage the area if the inflammation is caused by a recent injury, or is accompanied by heat, redness, or pain.

MASSAGE FOR ARTHRITIS

Arthritis is a painful condition of the joints, where inflammation causes discomfort and lessens mobility. Massage can help to reduce muscle tension and pain, lessen stiffness, and increase mobility. Massage also eases anxiety and can help promote more restful sleep (see here).

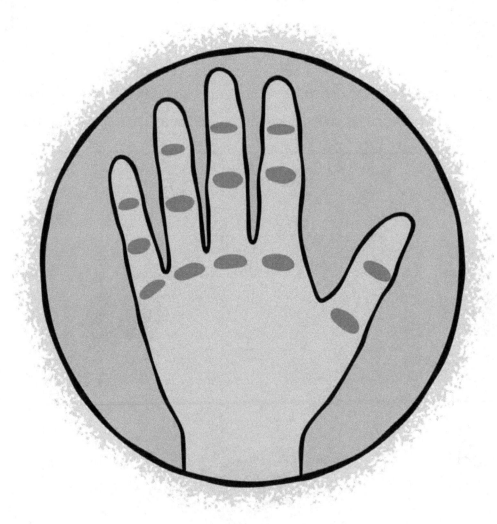

Method

When massaging a person with arthritis, the most important thing to bear in mind is communication: everyone has a different level of pain tolerance, and it is important to work within the threshold of the receiver. Massage should never feel painful or irritating.

To massage an area of arthritic discomfort, begin with gentle **compression**.

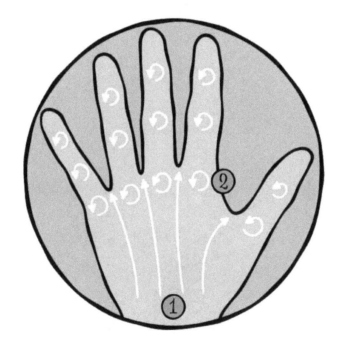

① For **effleurage**, focus on lighter work with long, gliding strokes. Deeper work is not helpful because it can cause extra soreness.

② You can also use light to medium **circular petrissage** strokes on the affected areas. Always proceed with caution, and if an area feels sensitive, be sure to avoid it.

6 SELF-MASSAGE

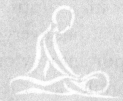

Take care of your body. It's the only place you have to live.

JIM ROHN

HAND TECHNIQUES

Self-massage is a convenient way to treat your own pain or discomfort, when you need to. You can use relaxed hands, elbows, and forearms to apply pressure to areas in need of massage, making sure to avoid any unnecessary tension in other areas. Keep your shoulders relaxed and breathe deeply as you work on yourself.

Head

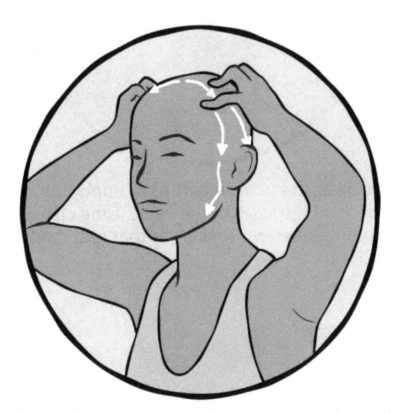

Using your fingertips, travel from the top of your head down to the sides of your temples, focusing on the area in front of and behind the ears. Continue to travel down the sides of your face into your jaw, noticing any adhesions or areas of tension, and pressing slowly and deeply until they release.

Neck

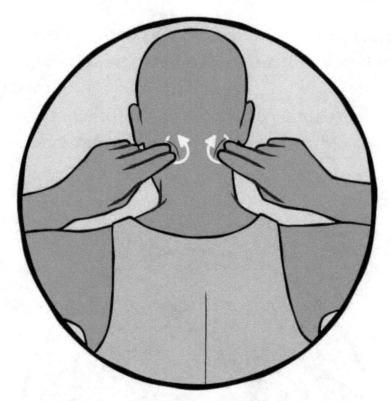

To massage the neck, use your fingertips to apply compression to the points of tension on the sides of the neck, using circular friction to explore adhesions and areas that feel tender.

Forearms

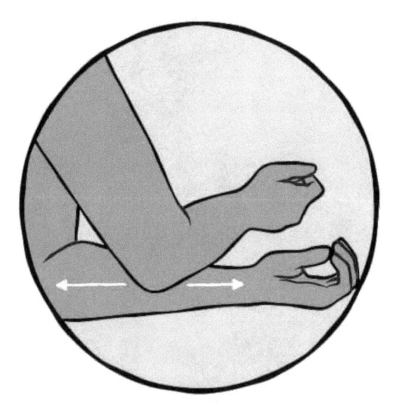

Apply oil and warm up the receiving arm using a long, gliding effleurage stroke. Rest the arm on a surface and use the opposite forearm to apply slow and steady pressure, working up from elbow to wrist and back down again. This is a lovely and easy way to work on your arms after a day of typing (or massaging)!

Pectoral muscles

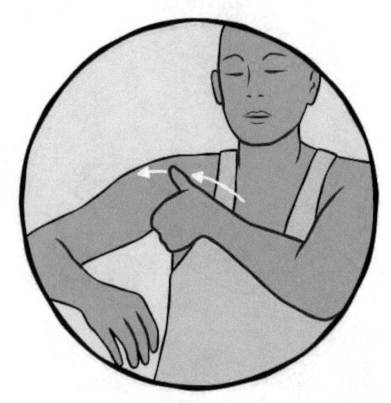

Apply oil and warm up the area using long, gliding effleurage strokes. Make slow, circular strokes along the pectoral muscle, starting at the sternum or breastbone, and moving out toward the shoulder where the muscle attaches. Work more deeply by pinching the muscle between your thumb and fingers. Use your fingers to scoop up the belly of the muscle next to the underarm, and pin it between thumb and fingers (above). Use gentle, kneading petrissage strokes to address this area.

Feet

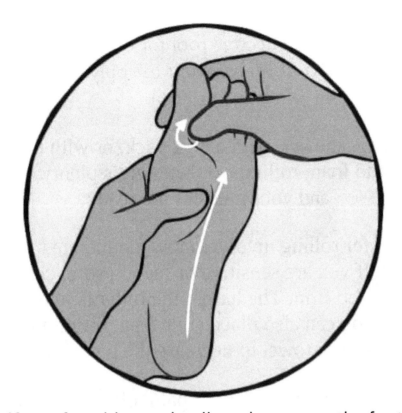

Seat yourself comfortably, apply oil, and warm up the foot using long, gliding effleurage strokes. Use a kneading petrissage stroke from heal to toe along the arch of the foot (above). Use your fingers to slowly roll your toes and provide a little traction or gentle pull (above). Use a fist to work under the foot. Hold the heel in the palm of your hand and move in a circular motion to stretch and mobilize your ankle. Don't forget to also work along the top of the foot, in between the toes, and along the length of the foot.

USING A FOAM ROLLER

A foam roller is a very effective tool for deep stretching and self-massage as it utilizes your bodyweight to apply pressure to different areas in need.

Warm up in the shower, with a heat pack, or with brisk physical activity prior to foam rolling, so that there's plenty of circulation and your muscles are ready.

The technique for rolling involves slow, deliberate movement over broad areas. If you are sensitive or feeling sore, choose a foam roller that isn't too firm. The harder the roller is, the more pressure you will feel. You can also place your foam roller on top of a yoga mat or towel to decrease the pressure.

Always work within your level of pain tolerance. Hold each area for a few long breaths as you slowly roll your body over the foam roller, easing it into areas that feel tight or restricted.

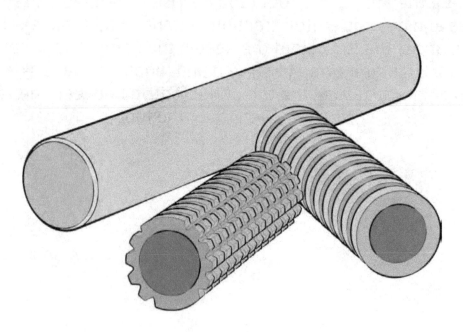

Pectoral muscles

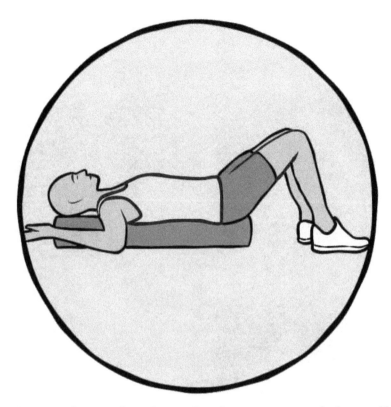

With your knees bent, lay lengthwise on top of the roller, firmly planting your feet for balance. To stretch your chest, allow your arms to fall to the sides, opening up the rib cage as you inhale deeply.

Upper back

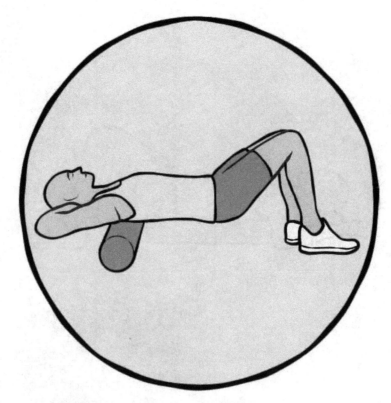

Position the roller widthwise under your upper back and slowly roll up and down, breathing deeply into areas of tension. For deeper pressure, cross your arms in front of your chest in a hugging position.

Hips

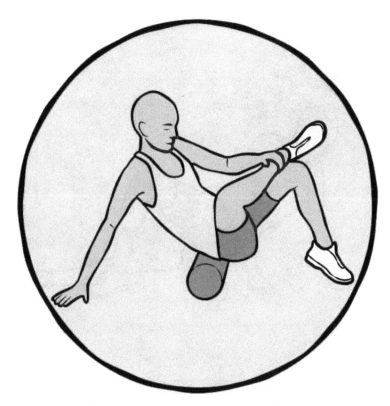

Start seated on the roller, crossing your ankle over the opposite knee. Lean your body toward the side of your hip to target the deep hip muscles. Roll slowly back and forth, pausing over areas of discomfort or tension until you feel the muscles release.

IT band

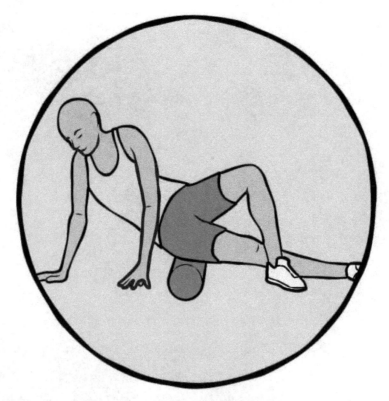

Lay on your side and position the roller below your hip. Slowly roll from hip to knee. If you find this position too painful or intense, bend your top knee and plant your top foot on the ground for less pressure and more control. For increased pressure, keep your top leg straight.

Back of legs

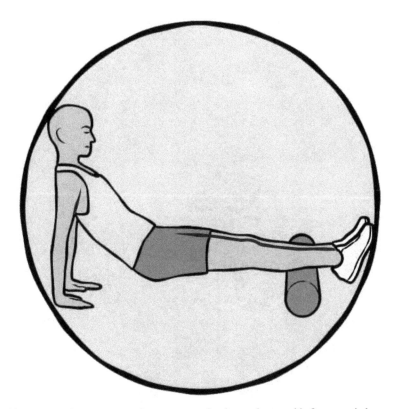

Place the roller under your legs and slowly roll from hip to ankle. You can increase the pressure on one leg at a time by crossing one ankle over the other.

Front of legs

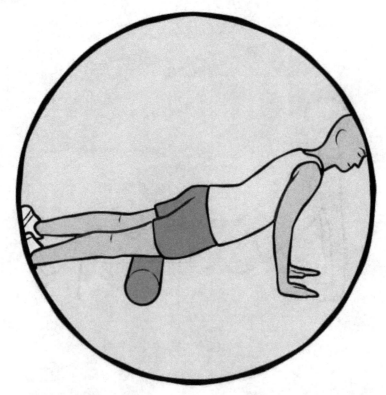

Lay face down with the roller underneath you at the top of your legs, and slowly roll down to the knees (do not roll over the knees). For increased pressure, cross one leg over the other.

USING A BALL

For deeper or more specific pressure, a tennis ball, squash ball, or even golf ball can be used for self-massage. Warm up the tissue with physical activity, a heat pack, or a long hot shower. Place the ball in an area of tension and use your bodyweight to apply pressure to that area. Slowly roll the ball over areas with adhesions. If you notice a trigger point, spend extra time in that area, breathing deeply into it.

Hips

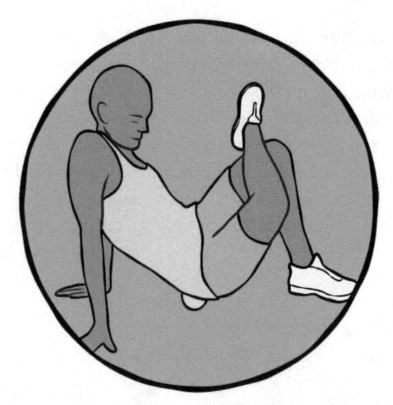

For deeply targeted pressure, cross one ankle over the opposite knee, placing the ball in the soft part of your gluteal muscles, avoiding any bones. Find a position that feels comfortable for you, and slowly adjust as needed.

Side of hip

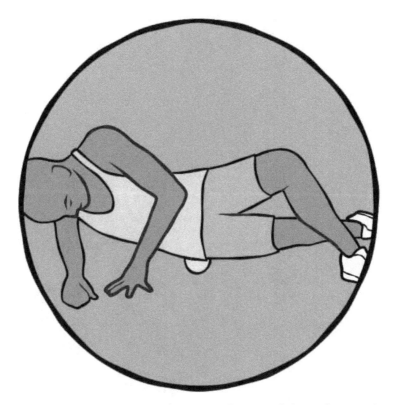

To address the muscles on the side of your hip, place the ball under the hip and use slow, deep compression.

Foot

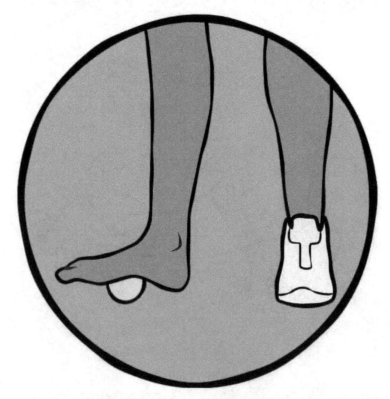

For a pain-relieving foot massage, try placing a ball under the arch of your foot and rolling slowly back and forth. Experiment with pressure by using different balls.

Shoulder

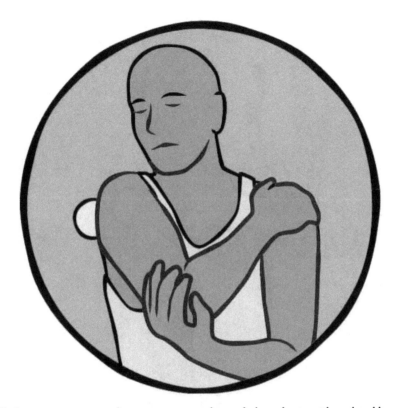

Using a wall for support, lean your shoulder into the ball, adjusting for pressure as needed. Move slowly and breathe deeply as the muscles release.

Upper shoulder

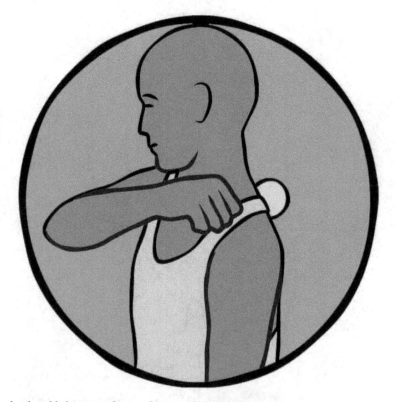

A single tennis ball is perfect for addressing the sore upper and middle trapezius muscles of the shoulder. Use a wall to lean into the ball and pause over areas of tension, releasing the muscles as you breathe deeply.

Neck

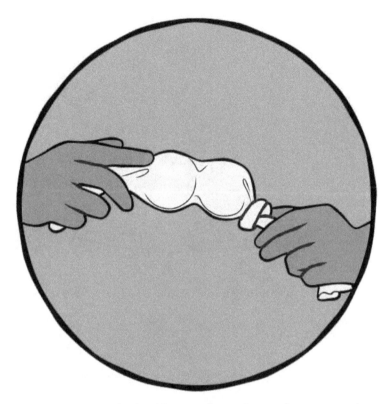

Fill a sock with two tennis balls and make a knot at the end (above). Lay flat on your back, allowing the weight of your head to apply pressure on the balls, gently moving them to areas of pain or tension.

Arm flexors

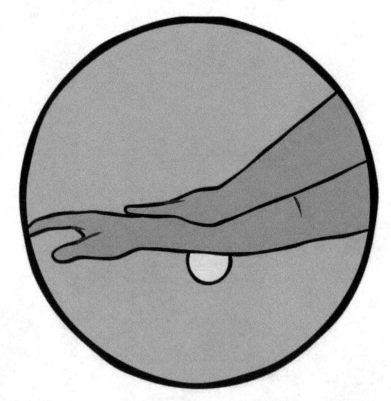

Place the ball on a flat surface, such as a table or desk, and slowly roll the ball along your arm and wrist. For additional depth, apply pressure with your top hand.

Arm extensors

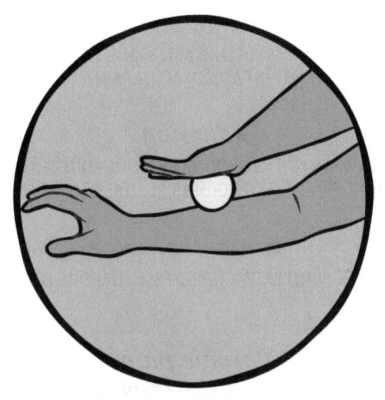

The most effective way to address the top of your arm is to use your opposite hand to guide the ball from elbow to wrist, increasing pressure as needed.

GLOSSARY

Acute pain

TEMPORARY, SUDDEN PAIN THAT OCCURS AFTER AN ACCIDENT OR INJURY. MASSAGE IS NOT APPROPRIATE IN CASES OF ACUTE PAIN.

Adhesion

KNOTS THAT FORM WHEN LAYERS OF MUSCLE BECOME ADHERED OR STUCK TO OVERLAYING OR UNDERLAYING STRUCTURES, SUCH AS OTHER MUSCLES.

Aromatherapy

THE USE OF AROMATIC PLANT EXTRACTS AND ESSENTIAL OILS TO PROMOTE HEALING.

Chronic pain

LONG-LASTING PAIN THAT RE-OCCURS. EXAMPLES INCLUDE REGULAR HEADACHES AND ARTHRITIS. MASSAGE MAY BE APPROPRIATE IN CASES OF CHRONIC PAIN.

Compression

RELAXING MASSAGE STROKE THAT INVOLVES USING THE FLAT PALMS OF THE HANDS TO GRADUALLY APPLY AND RELEASE PRESSURE OVER AN AREA.

Cross-fiber friction

A FIRM, DEEP MASSAGE STROKE PERFORMED ACROSS THE LENGTH OF A MUSCLE.

Effleurage

SMOOTH, GLIDING MASSAGE STROKE MADE WITH THE PALM OF THE HAND TO OPEN A SESSION AND INTRODUCE YOUR TOUCH TO THE RECEIVER. ALSO USED IN BETWEEN DEEPER STROKES TO CREATE FLOW.

Ergonomics

PRINCIPLES OF GOOD POSTURE AND METHODS OF WORKING TO MINIMIZE PAIN AND STRAIN INJURIES.

Hyper-irritable muscle

A BAND OF MUSCLE EXPERIENCING AN INVOLUNTARY CONTRACTION THAT CREATES REFERRED PAIN IN ANOTHER AREA OF THE BODY.

Knead

SEE PETRISSAGE.

Knots

SEE ADHESION.

Mobilize

SMALL PASSIVE MOVEMENTS, USUALLY APPLIED AS A SERIES OF GENTLE STRETCHES IN A SMOOTH, RHYTHMIC FASHION.

Muscular attachments

AREAS WHERE MUSCLES ATTACH TO THE BONE.

Petrissage

MEDIUM-PRESSURE MASSAGE STROKE THAT INVOLVES PICKING UP AND KNEADING THE MUSCLES.

Referred pain

PAIN FELT AT A LOCATION OTHER THAN THE SITE OF THE PAINFUL STIMULUS.

Stripping

THE APPLICATION OF SLOW, DEEP, GLIDING PRESSURE ALONG THE LENGTH OF THE MUSCLE FIBERS.

Swedish massage

A SERIES OF MASSAGE STROKES CREATED BY P. H. LING, INCLUDING EFFLEURAGE, PETRISSAGE, STRIPPNG, CROSS-FIBER FRICTION, COMPRESSION, AND TAPOTEMENT. USED FOR THE PURPOSE OF CREATING RELAXATION, RELIEVING PAIN AND TENSION, AND INCREASING CIRCULATION.

Tapotement

A RAPID AND REPEATED, LIGHT PUMMELING MASSAGE STROKE.

Tension

REFERS TO THE DISCOMFORT CREATED BY PROLONGED STRESS (PHYSICAL OR PSYCHOLOGICAL) WHICH IS FELT IN THE MUSCLE AS A SEMI-CONTRACTION.

Trigger points

COMMON HYPER-IRRITABLE BANDS OF MUSCLE THAT CONTAIN A CONTRACTION NODULE THAT CREATES A PAIN-REFERRAL PATTERN IN AN AREA FAR FROM THE AREA BEING COMPRESSED.

Wat Po School

TRAINING SCHOOL FOR THAI MASSAGE THERAPISTS AT THE WAT PO TEMPLE IN BANGKOK.

INDEX

Illustrations are in *italic*. Glossary words are in **bold**.

rosemary oil 37, 99

CPSIA information can be obtained
at www.ICGtesting.com
Printed in the USA
LVHW020752160322
713569LV00008B/667